CEREBRAL P[
PROBLEMS AND PRACTICE

HUMAN HORIZONS SERIES

CEREBRAL PALSY
Problems and Practice

Margaret Griffiths
and
Mary Clegg

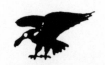

A CONDOR BOOK
SOUVENIR PRESS (E & A LTD)

First published 1988 by Souvenir Press (Educational &
    Academic) Ltd,
43 Great Russell Street, London WC1B 3PA
and simultaneously in Canada

ISBN 0 285 65066 1 hardback
ISBN 0 285 65071 8 paperback

Photoset in Great Britain by
Rowland Phototypesetting Ltd,
Bury St Edmunds, Suffolk
Printed in Great Britain by
St Edmundsbury Press Ltd,
Bury St Edmunds, Suffolk

Contents

Contents

Preface

There have been many changes in the services provided for disabled children during the past two decades. Medical and paramedical care have been greatly improved by closer contact between hospital and community staff, with involvement of other professionals and also, much more importantly, the parents. In the educational field the 1981 Education Act strongly recommends the admission of handicapped children to ordinary schools, giving parents a say in the 'Statement' which should decide their child's educational placement.

Because of the increasing number of children with cerebral palsy who will mix with normal peers and their families, and because teachers in ordinary schools will find in their classes increasing numbers of children with a bewildering variety of problems, this book is intended to offer an outline of the difficulties that these children encounter.

Parents and often teachers may well be confused to find that programmes designed for one child may not be appropriate for another. We have attempted to explain the reasons for the diversity encountered, and to outline most of the ways of support that are commonly used.

Detailed specific 'recipes' cannot be applied to a large group of children, such as are considered in the book, which is based on our experience mainly in the West Midlands, and especially in the Community Health Services and Children's Unit in Dudley. Further information can be obtained from use of the Reference sections at the end of each chapter.

We are very grateful to all our colleagues and to our patients who have taught us so much. Our particular thanks go to those young people who have made their own, very special, contributions.

Mrs Kathleen Burston has typed the manuscript with patience and efficiency. The sketches in Figures 1–39 were produced by Sarah Denvir and the photographs by A. J. Coote of Dudley Health Authority.

Margaret Griffiths
Mary Clegg

Part One

THE BACKGROUND

Formulating the Problem

1 What is Cerebral Palsy?

I keep six honest serving men
(They taught me all I knew)
Their names are What and Why and When
And How and Where and Who

Rudyard Kipling

What?

Cerebral palsy is a phrase describing certain conditions of difficulty in movement encountered in childhood. Owing to its diversity and complexity it has never been easy to find a simple definition, indeed Scrutton (1984) wrote 'The almost infinite variety (and the lack of a common language to describe this variety accurately) makes learning about it very difficult indeed.'

In view of the fact that we are confronting difficulties both of language and understanding, it seems wise to use the most comprehensive and authoritative definition available. This comes from the World Commission for Cerebral Palsy and states that cerebral palsy is 'a persistent but not unchanging disorder of movement and posture due to dysfunction of the brain, excepting that caused by progressive disease, present before its growth and development are completed. Many other clinical signs may be present.'

This somewhat daunting sentence expresses the complexity and diversity of the ways in which children may be affected by the condition of cerebral (from the brain) palsy (difficulty of movement). However, to be useful this definition needs to be expanded into a narrative form.

Persistent means that cerebral palsy is lifelong. It cannot be 'cured' although, as it is *not unchanging*, development, maturation and intervention may alter the movement patterns.

Disorder of movement and posture is reflected in difficulty in control of movement and of position at rest. These difficulties may be apparent in any part of the body; may exist as stiffness or unwanted movements; and are exacerbated by lack of control of the rest of the body (*disorder of posture*), making intentional movements less attainable.

The *dysfunction of the brain* may be due to a variety of influences, (*excepting that caused by progressive disease*). The location within the brain will determine the type of disorder of movement and posture, the parts of the body which are affected and also whether other neurological functions are impaired and to what extent (thus *many other clinical signs may be present*).

Because the dysfunction of the brain is *present before its growth and development are completed* the characteristics of the motor disorder may alter during this period, and indeed may not be apparent during the first few months of life.

Why?

Dysfunction of the brain may be ascribed to many causes. In cerebral palsy progressive disease is specifically excluded; the brain impairment, once it has occurred, can be expected to remain static and changes in its effects are due to maturation and development.

Impairment leading to dysfunction may be inherited or acquired after conception. Inherited cases are thought to be very rare, probably less than one per cent (Bundey and Griffiths, 1977). Cerebral palsy is usually the result of some hazard adversely affecting the brain some time after conception, around birth or during childhood.

The question Why? may have different implications. 'Why does it happen?' considers statistics in a population with the purpose of seeking ways to prevent recurrences, and of planning future services. 'Why did it happen to me/him/her?' is more personal and equally important. Parents and child need to know, so that particular care may be taken to eliminate specific risks in future pregnancies; the future for siblings and for grandchildren can be fully discussed; professionals involved together with parents may plan individual programmes; prospects for the child's future may be more accurately predicted.

When?

By definition the dysfunction of the brain which leads to cerebral palsy occurs during its development, and so it will be helpful to consider the normal sequence.

The single cell formed at conception by the fusion of the mother's ovum and the father's sperm, divides very rapidly and by 14 days after conception cells that will form the central nervous system can be found as a ridge on the back of the embryo. This then forms a tube extending from head to tail. By the end of the fourth week, three pouches are formed at the head end, and these will become the three parts of the brain. From this time onwards a central area of the future brain produces new cells (neurons) which migrate to various parts of the brain where they acquire specific functions.

All neurons have the same basic structure (see Figure 1) (Mellor, 1985), although in migrating to various locations in the brain they acquire their special functions and some-times individual structural characteristics. The neurons which are to perform specific functions are all present by the 25th week of pregnancy and no more will be produced. From this time onwards growth of the brain is due to the formation of new connecting cells, with further develop-ment of dendrites, and the growth and thickening of myelin sheaths around the axons. This process continues after the baby is born, certainly until the end of his second year, and to a smaller extent until he is five. By then the skull ceases to grow, although activity within the brain continues to progress for the rest of life, bringing more dormant specialist neurons into use, and improving the network of communications and the speed of transmission of more complex messages.

This understanding of the pattern of brain development has certain important implications for the nature of cerebral palsy and the ways in which its effects may be mitigated:

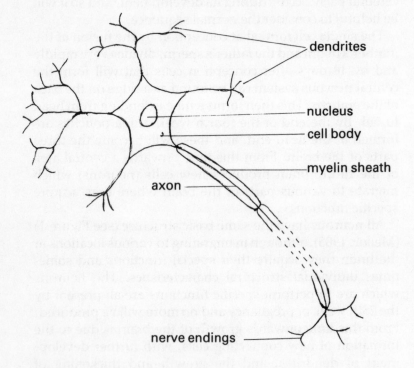

Notes
Cell body may have various shapes
Nucleus controls the function of the neuron
Axon may be long or short
Myelin sheath increases with the work of the axon and
determines the speed of conduction of impulses.

Fig. 1   A neuron.

1) The special action of different neurons in their allotted locations in the brain, means that other, undamaged, parts cannot take over the function of damaged areas; 2) The continuing development of connections between neurons and the improvement in communications by increasing use of axons and dendrites, emphasises the importance of encouraging such development by carefully devised programmes of therapy and education; 3) The times of the hazard experienced will affect the nature of the brain impairment and the disability experienced by the child; 4) The When, the How, and the Where are factors that are mutually interdependent.

There are certain definite periods which can be expected to throw up risks to the child and particularly the brain.

a)   Prenatal (From conception to birth)
During the first 13 weeks as an embryo, severe hazards may cause miscarriage. If less severe or in the 13–25 weeks before the brain is fully differentiated, the production of neurons may be limited and the brain (and sometimes the baby) may be smaller than it should be, with resulting mental impairment and in some cases cerebral palsy. The third trimester (26–40 weeks) of pregnancy is usually relatively free of risk unless the mother has high blood pressure, the placenta fails, or the baby is born prematurely.
b)   Premature delivery (26–36 weeks)
This is still one of the puzzles of human development. Some of these babies are 'small-for-dates' and it may be that they have suffered some form of disadvantage in the uterus which has caused the premature delivery, i.e. a prenatal hazard which may already have caused impairment of brain function. Others are 'appropriate-for-dates', small healthy babies whose potential for development can be expected to be normal provided that their lungs, liver and heart are enabled to perform the life-giving functions which would normally come into action at full term.
c)   Perinatal (During labour and delivery)
Careful surveillance during pregnancy can be expected to

reduce the risks to the minimum, but emergencies may occur, and skilled specialist care should always be available if needed.

d)   Neonatal (0–28 days)

Hazards in the prenatal or perinatal period, and prematurity may lead to the need for skilled professional care for the baby in a Special Care Baby Unit or, in a few very complex cases, in an Intensive Care Unit. It is usually said that the best time to transfer a baby for special care is while still in utero, and most babies who have given due warning of difficulties ahead will be delivered in a hospital where facilities are available for treating babies who are at risk. However, it may become necessary to transfer a few babies after they are born.

e)   Post-natal (One month and onwards)

Although only a small proportion (approximately five per cent) of children who have cerebral palsy acquire it at an older age, infections and accidents (in the home, at school or on holiday, or on the roads) may cause severe handicap.

How?

The multiplication, growth and survival of living cells throughout the body depends upon an adequate and balanced supply of oxygen, nutriments (both general and special for particular functions) and necessary hormones. The cells in the brain are sensitive to these needs. Oxygen is the most important, as without it cells will cease to function and will ultimately die. Cells may also be affected by chemical and biochemical substances not normally present (or present in grossly increased quantity), and by living organisms. Impairment may occur at any stage in brain development and the time at which it occurs has a direct relationship with the type of impairment produced.

During the prenatal period the placenta is the source of all supplies to and the removal of waste products from the foetus. Through it oxygen is diffused from the maternal to the foetal red blood cells and deficiency of oxygen (hypoxia) may be caused by a poor supply from the mother, or by an inefficient placenta. All nutrients are selectively supplied in suitable form, such as glucose and amino acids, together with hormones and enzymes which the brain needs and which the foetus is not yet producing in sufficient quantity. It normally acts as a barrier to toxic substances (although nicotine, alcohol and hard drugs can get through) and infections (although viruses and some other organisms can penetrate).

After premature delivery the brain is at risk—something may have gone wrong prenatally to cause the prematurity; the baby may suffer from hypoxia because the lungs are not fully expanding or the heart is not functioning as it should; hypoxia may affect the function of the nerve cells directly or may cause local haemorrhage by damaging the fine capillary blood vessels supplying the brain (this is thought to be a possible cause of spastic diplegia, see pp. 32–5); temperature changes may interfere with the ability of cells to utilise oxygen and nutrients; jaundice due to the excessive breakdown of red blood cells may cause damage to cells in the basal ganglia (which may be a cause of athetosis, see pp. 36–41).

Birth is a journey in which, as in other kinds of travel, forseeable hazards have usually been reduced to a minimum, particularly when prenatal care has been of a high standard. However, even in the best circumstances something may go wrong at the last moment, leading to trauma or hypoxia, and some full term babies may need special care during the first week of life.

Neonatal problems follow prenatal, premature or perinatal hazards. There may be hypoxia, hypoglycaemia (low blood sugar) or other less common biochemical disturbances, or convulsions which may or may not indicate serious difficulty. Modern methods of treating breathing problems by intubation, and of metabolic (body chemistry) disturbances by suitable drip treatment have increased the chances of survival of children cared for in Special Care Units, but may also contribute to the number of survivors who have cerebral palsy (Hagberg, 1982).

Post-natal disasters only contribute about five per cent of children who have cerebral palsy but it is usually severe. Causes may be apnoea (lack of breathing) associated with urgent operations or epileptic status, infections of the brain which do not respond to treatment or head injury from accidents in the home (including non-accidental injury), in playgrounds or road accidents.

Although knowledge of ways of prevention of cerebral palsy is increasing, so also are the possible hazards, so that it is not surprising that cerebral palsy is still a significant part of handicap in childhood.

Where?

In a child who has cerebral palsy any of the three areas in the brain which participate in the control of movement and posture may be affected, and the location of these motor cells determines the type of disorder that ensues. The

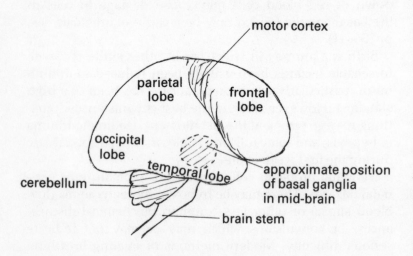

Locations of motor neurons

Fig. 2   Surface view of the right side of the brain.

location of impairment in the brain is closely reflected in the child, both in the parts of the body that are affected and the type of difficulty experienced (Figure 2) (Mellor, 1985).

The cells in the *motor cortex* of each cerebral hemisphere control the opposite side of the body and are responsible for conscious voluntary movements. All parts of the body are mapped out in detail in the distribution of the cells, and the intricate movements for manipulation and speech are generously represented. The axons from the cells, which control the trunk and limbs, extend into the spinal cord and activate or inhibit the cells there which form the nerves going to individual muscles. For control of eyes, tongue, face and palate the axons are much shorter and terminate at nuclei in the brain stem. Impairment of functions may result from damage to the cell body of the neuron or to its axon within the brain.

The difficulty in movement which is caused by interference with these pathways is known as *spasticity* and is characterised by a particular kind of stiffness and slowing of movement.

Because of the wide representation of motor cells in the cortex of both cerebral hemispheres, spasticity may sometimes be limited to one half of the body (spastic hemiplegia) or the legs alone (spastic diplegia), however, all four limbs may be involved (spastic tetraplegia/quadriplegia).

The conscious voluntary efforts inaugurated by the motor cortex need further controls. The neurons in the *basal ganglia* are responsible for 'tone' and posture throughout the body, keeping head, trunk and limbs in the best positions relative to gravity. Impairment in this area causes flailing and jerky movements (*athetosis*) and sometimes immobility and stiffness (*dystonia*). The *cerebellum* co-ordinates the actions of groups of muscles and is responsible for *balance*; impairment of these functions causes unsteadiness, staggering and shaky movements. The very compact accumulation of cells in the basal ganglia and cerebellum means that interference at these locations usually affects all four limbs.

Eye movements, swallowing, chewing and speech may be affected in any of these conditions.

Functions in other parts of the brain may also be affected if the disturbance is widespread or the cells are particularly susceptible to its influence. Some of these other functions directly affect the ability to control and direct movement. In this respect the most important are the feedback mechanisms from tendons and joints, which inform the motor neurons at a subconscious level of the tension in muscles and the position of joints. Thus the maintenance of posture and the activation of movements are subject to a very complex system of computerised control within the brain.

In addition, the conditions which have impaired the functions of direct motor control in the brain, may lead to interference with other important contributory activities. Vision, hearing, all aspects of the learning process, attention and alertness, may be impaired and centres of scarring may become the focus for epilepsy.

Who?
From the time of conception until the end of our life, we all have to face hazards of varying degrees of complexity. When we are older, we take all sorts of precautions: we have immunisations; we look to safety in our homes, our cars, on public transport; we take out insurances. The embryo and foetus have to take what comes, and although the mother may take every precaution she knows and will look after herself for the sake of her child, a variety of hazards already described may overtake them both. From available statistics around the world most countries can expect that approximately two out of every 1000 liveborn will have cerebral palsy (Paneth and Kiely, 1984).

Although it is possible to define characteristics of groups of children at greatest risk, it is impossible to formulate a simple answer concerning individuals.

In almost all developed countries and many in the Third World, perinatal and infant mortality is declining and the incidence of cerebral palsy to some extent is declining with it, but very much less rapidly, and in many countries it is stationary. Since 1862 when Little drew attention to the effects of 'abnormal parturition, difficult labours, premature birth and asphyxia neonatorum, on the mental and physical condition of the child' many of the hazards of the perinatal period have been identified and, to a large extent, prevented. However, very often, a decline in one group of children is matched by an increase in another. Reports in the 1970s and 1980s provide a more up-to-date picture of the present situation.

Stanley (1979) in Western Australia and Hagberg and his colleagues (1975) in Sweden demonstrated a fall in the incidence of cerebral palsy in the bigger babies, but an increased survival in low birth-weight babies was accompanied by an increase in cerebral palsy in this group, leaving the overall figures almost unchanged. The decrease in numbers in the heavier babies is thought to be due to better social conditions, good maternal health and to a lesser extent improved prenatal and obstetric care. In the case of the smaller babies (1000–1500 gms) special care has become more widely used and is a subject of careful study throughout the world. The value of very intensive care for very small, or sickly, newborns has been questioned in some quarters. All recent reports concerned with the future for low birth-weight babies (Kitchen et al, 1979; Dale and Stanley, 1980; Hagberg et al, 1982) have shown a fall in mortality with an increased incidence of cerebral palsy. However, Hagberg makes the point that 'considerable net "gain" in the number of lives saved without cerebral palsy has been achieved.' All these workers point to the need to identify any additional factors which may be the precipitating cause of cerebral palsy in some individuals, and in particular what unidentified prenatal factors might be involved.

The position remains that despite all known preventive measures and increasing skills in producing and keeping babies alive, a small number will have cerebral palsy. Although some risk factors are well known, it is impossible at present to identify the most vulnerable children amongst the groups.

References

BUNDEY, S. and GRIFFITHS, M. (1977). 'Recurrence risks in families of Children with cerebral palsy', *Developmental Medicine and Child Neurology*, **19**, 179–191.

DALE, A. and STANLEY, F. (1980). 'An epidemiological study of cerebral palsy in Western Australia 1956–1975'. *Developmental Medicine and Child Neurology*, **22**, 13–25.

HAGBERG, B., HAGBERG, G. and OLOW, I. (1975). 'The changing panorama of cerebral palsy in Sweden, 1954–1970. I. Analysis of the general changes', *Acta Paediatrica Scandinavica*, **64**, 187–192.

HAGBERG, B., HAGBERG, G. and OLOW, I. (1982). 'Gains and hazards of intensive neonatal care: an analysis from Swedish cerebral palsy epidemiology', *Developmental Medicine and Child Neurology*, **24**, 13–19.

KITCHEN, W. H., RICKARDS, A., RYAN, M. M., McDOUGALL, A. B., BILLSON, F. A., KEIR, E. H. and NAYLOR, F. D. (1979). 'A longitudinal study of very low-birthweight infants. II: Results of controlled trial of intensive care and incidence of handicaps', *Developmental Medicine and Child Neurology*, **21**, 582–589.

LITTLE, W. J. (1862). 'On the influence of abnormal parturition, difficult labours, premature birth and asphyxia neonatorum, on the mental and physical condition of the child especially in relation to deformities', *Obstetrical Transactions*, **3**, 293.

MELLOR, D. (1985). 'How the brain works', in *Working Together with Handicapped Children*, pp. 60–83. GRIFFITHS, M. and RUSSELL, P. (eds). London: Souvenir Press.

PANETH, N. and KIELY, J. (1984). 'The frequency of cerebral palsy: a review of population studies in industrialised nations since 1950', in *The Epidemiology of the Cerebral Palsies*, pp. 46–56. STANLEY, F. and ALBERMAN, E. (eds). Spastics International Medical Publications; Oxford: Blackwell; Philadelphia: Lippincott.

SCRUTTON, D. (1984). 'Aim-oriented management', in *Management of the Motor Disorders in Cerebral Palsy*. pp. 49–58.

SCRUTTON, D. (ed). Spastics International Medical Publications; Oxford: Blackwell; Philadelphia: Lippincott.
STANLEY, F. J. (1979). 'An epidemiological study of cerebral palsy in Western Australia, 1956–1975. I. Changes in total incidence of cerebral palsy and associated factors', *Developmental Medicine and Child Neurology*, **21**, 701–713.

2   Children Who Have Cerebral Palsy

Our bodies why do we forbear?
They're ours, though they're not we, we are
The intelligences, they the sphere

John Donne

This chapter is to consider children, reminding ourselves that just as ordinary children, even children in one family, differ from one another, so children who have cerebral palsy show even greater differences amongst themselves.

Moreover, to take up the quotation above, it is children as individual personalities, over and above their physical problems, with whom we are concerned. All children need love, security and encouragement in developing their abilities, thoughts and feelings, but children who have additional problems need something more. To give them this extra support we must understand their needs, and for that reason it is necessary to discern the specific difficulties in each individual child.

1.   Problems of Movement
Normal patterns
The way in which the brain controls movement was outlined very briefly in Chapter 1. In a young child this control of movement is developed gradually as the brain matures and the various areas in it are able to take up their allotted functions; until this has happened the child's ability to undertake skilled voluntary movement is limited. As this control, much of it subconscious, is developed the child is able to react and interact with his surroundings. Movement is rarely an end in itself but a response to a variety of stimuli: turning to a known voice, smiling at a known face, reaching out for an attractive object, changing position and place to explore and to obtain. While this is going on the child is also exploring his own body, watching his hands, putting them in his mouth, finding his toes, making his own noises, and discovering all sorts of ways to move about. Although the

baby and his observers may not realise it, this is all according to a pattern of development programmed in the brain, which synchronises not only the development of the threefold control of movement, but also the development of seeing and hearing, of sense of position in space, of the meaning of objects (mother's face, pram, cot, toys, food, etc.) and of the formation of relationships.

During the first three to four months babies are not wholly motionless but their movements at this time are not entirely voluntary. These movements are largely due to the persistence of primitive reflexes which initiate whole body movements, thought to be possibly vestigial automatic reactions remaining from our evolutionary past relating to survival, but not appropriate to the development of full voluntary control. The more important of these are: the 'startle' reaction (Moro) which happens when the baby's head goes back, then the arms and hands shoot out and very rapidly bend in again, the fingers making a firm grasp; the 'ATNR' (asymmetric tonic neck reflex), a complex description of a complex reaction which is shown when the baby turns his head to one side, the arm and leg on that side shoot out whilst the arm and leg on the opposite side bend up; the 'grasp' reflex occurs when a finger is put on the baby's palm, it is immediately grasped and the baby is unable to let go; the 'stepping' reflex, when the baby is held up under his armpits with his toes on a firm surface, he makes stepping movements.

Voluntary motor control develops from above downwards beginning with the head, and is first seen when the baby, lying on his tummy, can turn the head to one side, and then hold it up for a short time when looking forwards, or can hold it up without support when picked up. Eventually the head can be held up in all positions of the body. Spinal control then assumes importance when the baby, lying on his back, starts to play with his hands and to kick his legs independently (Fig. 3). At the same time he is able to make rotational movements of his spine which will soon lead to rolling over (Figs 4 and 5), the beginning of

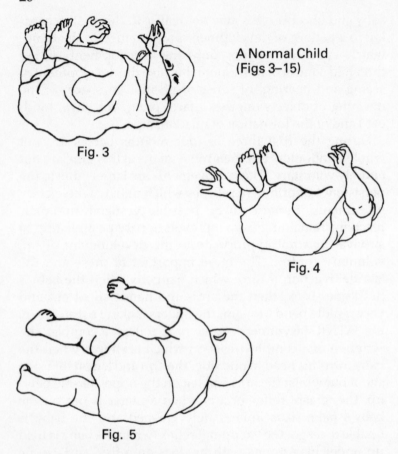

A Normal Child
(Figs 3–15)

Fig. 3

Fig. 4

Fig. 5

Rolling Over (Figs 3–5)

Fig. 3   This normal baby, when lying on his back, is able to keep his back firmly on the surface on which he is lying and bring his hand and feet up to touch and play where he can see them. He is also able to turn his head to a visual or auditory stimulus.

Fig. 4   This turning on the head will lead to turning onto his side and eventually rolling right over. The body will follow the head turning. The hand on the side to which he turns goes out to help . . .

Fig. 5   . . . and the legs straighten out to enable him to arrive flat on his tummy.

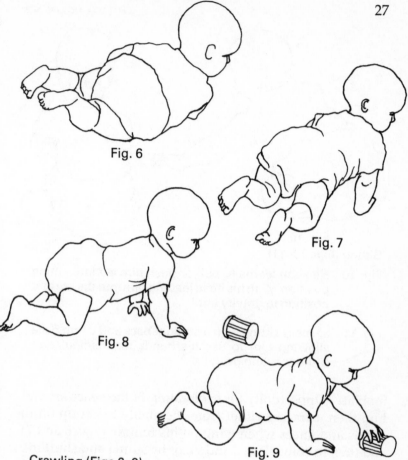

Fig. 6

Fig. 7

Fig. 8

Fig. 9

Crawling (Figs 6–9)

Fig. 6 From the position in Fig. 5 he lifts his head up when on his tummy, frees his arms to push up on his hands, bends his knees, and . . .

Fig. 7 . . . gets up to crawl.

Fig. 8 He can then crawl towards something which attracts his attention, with his head up, his eyes watching, his whole body posture happily secure and adjusting to gravity.

Fig. 9 With this stability he is able to support himself, and reach out with his hand to touch the toy which his eyes have seen—eye/hand control.

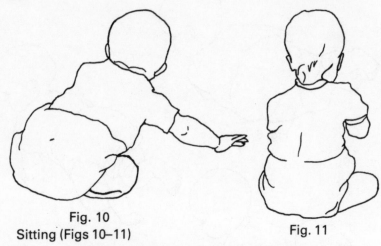

Fig. 10
Sitting (Figs 10–11)   Fig. 11

Fig. 10   He soon learns to pull or push himself into sitting
           position. With his head leading him into the upright
           position to gravity until . . .

Fig. 11   . . . he is sitting with a straight back and a firm base
           allowing him to use his hands for manipulation
           without falling over.

mobility. Opportunity for exploration of the space around
him then increases either from the ability to get up on to
hands and knees when lying on his tummy (Figs 6 and 7)
and then to crawl (Figs 8 and 9), or by sitting and shuffling
on his bottom, a method of getting about used by about 15
per cent of children (Robson, 1970). Soon afterwards he can
hold up his back without support and with the development of balance reactions is able to sit alone, thus freeing
his arms for independent use of his hands (Figs 10 and 11).

Once one or other method of moving around has been
achieved, the child begins to find that he can pull himself
up on to his feet by grasping any firm object (Figs 12, 13 and
14) and even before he can stand alone he will cruise around
the furniture (Fig. 15). Once full standing balance has been
acquired, he can then begin to transfer his weight over his
centre of gravity and find that he is able to take a few steps
alone. When this is accomplished, running, jumping and

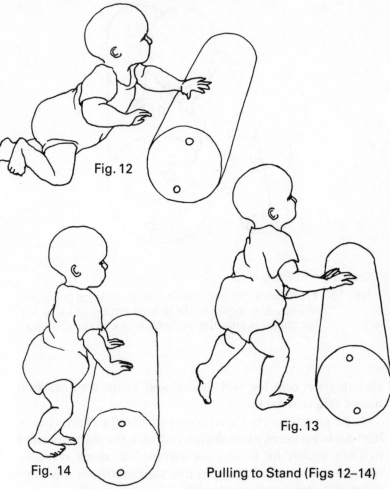

Fig. 12

Fig. 14   Fig. 13

Pulling to Stand (Figs 12–14)

Fig. 12   He can then begin to use his hands to pull himself to
stand. His head is up, and supporting himself on his
left knee and hand, he bends his right knee and
brings up the foot . . .

Fig. 13   . . . with his weight on both hands and his right foot,
he gets himself into standing . . .

Fig. 14   . . . firmly on two feet. His body weight automati-
cally adjusts itself to finding his centre of gravity
—usually somewhere around his hips.

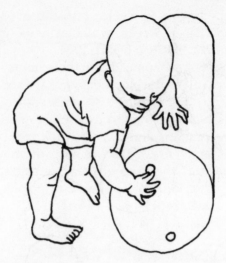

Cruising and Exploring
Fig. 15   From here, he can move about, holding onto the
           object, and explore. He is firm enough to use his
           hands for manipulation before he can stand alone.

standing on one leg will follow and more sophisticated
motor skills can be learnt.

As he progresses to the upright position the child's use of
his hands becomes more skilful and with the improvement
in near vision he is able to accomplish more complex
manual tasks, contributing in this way to further development of manual and social skills.

The importance for the human of the ability to walk is not
for its intrinsic value as a method of locomotion, which is
poor in contrast to that of most other mammals, but because
it frees both hands for manipulation in movement, greatly
improves the scope of communication and development of
social skills and reinforces curiosity and inventiveness in
the exploration of the surroundings.

Attainment of motor skills is achieved within a very wide
age range e.g. rolls over between 19 and 36 weeks, sits

alone (one minute) 24–36 weeks, cruising 33–52 weeks, pulling to stand 34–54 weeks, walks alone 50–75 weeks. (From Bower, 1977. See also Levitt, 1984.)

It is important to have some idea of these limits, although the normality of motor development is related more to the pattern of movements, regulated by maturation of an intact central nervous system, than to the timing. These can be accelerated by practice and may be delayed by causes outside the motor system by lack of motivation caused by poor vision, mental handicap or, very occasionally, limitations in the environment. The same principles apply to manipulation and speech as well as walking.

Patterns in cerebral palsy

In children who have cerebral palsy the acquisition of movement skills is invariably slower and their pattern is different. Technically these characteristics are referred to as delay and deviance.

Delay   During the first few months of life it is often difficult to be certain whether a baby thought to be at risk of developing cerebral palsy is affected. Much of the movement made by babies at this stage is a continuation of the reflex kicking and other movements that occurred before birth, and the automatic evolutionary primitive reactions. Some severely affected babies may have very limited movements, or feel very floppy or very stiff. It may not be until the early voluntary movements such as smiling, holding up the head or reaching for objects fail to occur that suspicion may be aroused or confirmed. In less severe conditions, especially when a child had not been considered at risk, it may be even longer before a diagnosis of cerebral palsy is made, although most children whose difficulty derives from around the time of birth are detected by one year of age. As the developmental skill expected becomes more complex the delay becomes more obvious.

Deviance   Cerebral palsy is always characterised by movement patterns that are different from the normal. This may in part be due to the persistence of primitive automatic reactions but the main characteristics will be due to the site of the brain dysfunction which determines the part of the body affected and the type of the change in movement, the difficulties that the child experiences reflecting the impairment in the brain, according to the three locations for control.

Spasticity is the commonest motor disorder, occurring in about 75 per cent, hence the choice of the name The Spastics Society in its concern for all children who have cerebral palsy. It is characterised by increased tension in muscles which are put on stretch or into action and which have difficulty in relaxing. Since all movements depend upon contraction and relaxation as required of the muscles concerned, in spasticity movements are slow, limited and stiff. Because some muscles are stronger than others and react more strongly against gravity or other forces, repeated wrong positions in movement or particularly at rest may cause deformities.

Because of the distribution of nerve cells in the motor cortex and the position of axonal tracts within the brain, it is possible for certain parts of the body to be affected on their own. In *spastic hemiplegia* one side only of the body is affected. The difficulty in movement is most obvious at first in the hand, and may only be manifest in the leg on weight bearing and walking. Due to unequal pull in the muscles the arm is often held in a typical position being pulled in at the shoulder, and bent at the elbow and wrist with the fist clenched. The gait is also affected, and is characterised by walking on the toes with a straight knee, and because there is a tendency to pull in at the hip, the leg is swung outwards and then inwards in a wide arc.

In *spastic diplegia* both legs are involved. Stiffness may be noticed early, particularly in separating the legs when changing nappies, and in rolling over. Ambulation is delayed and is characterised by walking on the toes with bent knees, the whole leg being pulled inwards with bent hips. The hands and arms are usually spared but there may be slight clumsiness and some difficulty in using eyes and

A Child with Spastic Diplegia
(Figs 16–23)

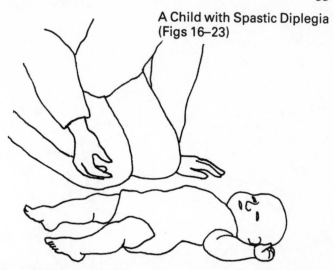

Fig. 16   With spasticity, stiffness in his legs and shoulders
will be noticed, especially when he is lying on his
back. This stiffness will prevent him from bringing
his feet and hands up to play as the normal baby
can (see Fig. 3).

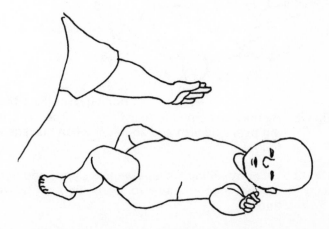

Fig. 17   It will also prevent his body from rolling over, even
when his head is turned (see Fig. 4).

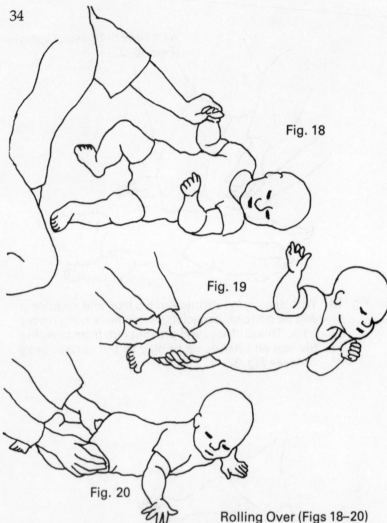

Fig. 18

Fig. 19

Fig. 20

Rolling Over (Figs 18–20)

Fig. 18   He may be helped to roll stiffly ... either by bringing over one arm and shoulder when his legs will
follow ...

Fig. 19   ... or by rolling his legs when his arms and hands
are left free for him to learn his own control,
thus ...

Fig. 20   ... he arrives safely on his tummy with his head
coming up to mid line, and his hands ready to try to
push himself up (see Figs 3–5 and 8–11).

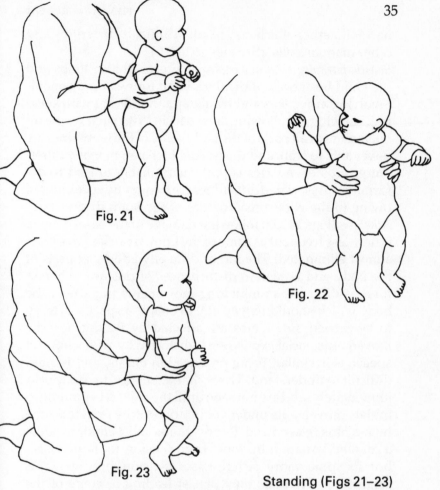

Fig. 21

Fig. 22

Fig. 23

Standing (Figs 21–23)

Fig. 21   This child is as yet unable to sit alone or to pull up to stand, and when put into standing he is unable to find his centre of gravity due to the absence of balance reactions and the spasticity which prevents his body adjusting.

Fig. 22   He may try to adjust and take a step by using his head and arms as well, but . . .

Fig. 23   . . . he finds as he tries to bend his leg the other one will not support him (see Figs 12–14 to compare the flexibility and adjustments in the normal child and the stiffness and instability in the spastic).

hands together which may result in difficulty in writing and other manual skills. (See Figs 16 to 23.)

Spastic tetraplegia (or quadriplegia) affects all four limbs and the child has severe difficulties in all forms of movement, involving arms, legs and trunk, and interfering with sucking, chewing, swallowing and speech. With such severe involvement of all parts of the body some of these children are never able to walk and the unequal tension in many different groups of muscles is particularly liable to lead to deformities. Associated difficulties are frequently encountered owing to the widespread nature of the brain dysfunction.

Athetosis (Figs 24–35) following damage to the basal ganglia is now less frequent as some of the known causes have been almost eliminated. The motor difficulty affects all parts of the body and is seen in disturbances of posture, wherein there is difficulty in inhibiting movements in parts of the body which should remain still to enable a specific activity to be carried out. Limbs are affected by flailing or jerky movements, facial expression is distorted by grimacing and speech is irregular, being produced in bursts, and is often difficult to understand. These characteristics do not appear immediately, and are not seen until the child is beginning to initiate movements under voluntary control; until this time he remains relaxed and 'floppy'. Later most children show a marked variation in 'tone' from tension to 'floppiness', but in some more severe cases tension prevails. This rigidity (or dystonia) may persist leading to some of the problems encountered in spasticity.

Ataxia is the least common form of motor difficulty occurring in less than ten per cent. It is characterised by continuing floppiness, tremor in the head and hands more marked with effort and an unsteadiness of gait, the child walking on a wide base and staggering at times. Speech may be affected and is typically monotone and staccato.

In all these descriptions of deviant motor patterns it needs to be stressed that a variety of movements may be restricted, and from the practical point of view this is what matters.

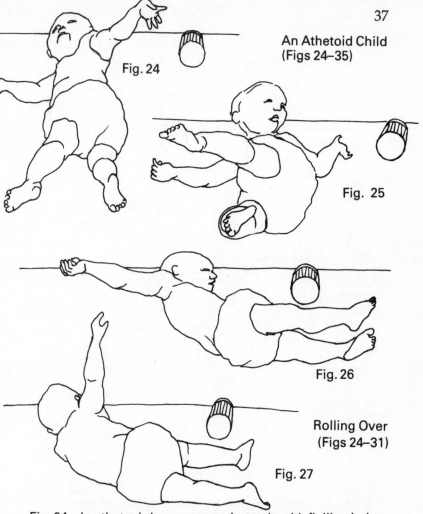

Fig. 24

Fig. 25

Fig. 26

Rolling Over
(Figs 24–31)

Fig. 27

Fig. 24   In athetosis he can move, but only with flailing jerky movements. As he tries to roll towards the toy, he starts the movement by turning his head, then flings his left arm over . . .

Fig. 25   . . . to bring himself onto his back, followed by straight stiff legs, which . . .

Fig. 26   . . . continue the movement over, with the right arm thrown out stiffly . . .

Fig. 27   . . . he manages to propel the arm over and . . .

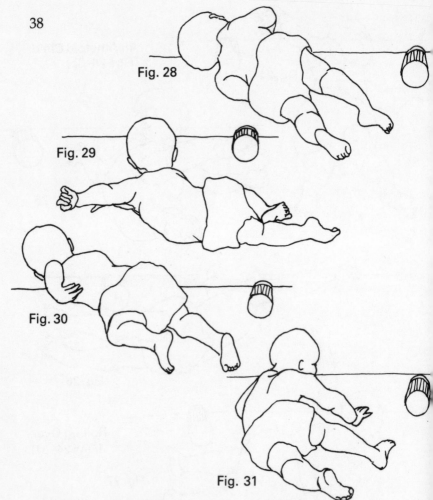

Fig. 28

Fig. 29

Fig. 30

Fig. 31

Fig. 28 . . . down. He then tries to bring the left arm out to push himself up but . . .

Fig. 29 . . . loses it as the elbow straightens.

Fig. 30 He then manages to rotate his pelvis and bends the left arm, bringing it up and . . .

Fig. 31 . . . underneath his body, thus enabling the right arm to push as he lifts his head to look towards the toy. The whole movement requires much effort and concentration on the part of the child and does not achieve its object (see Figs 3–5).

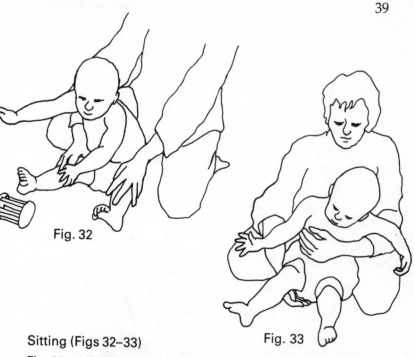

Fig. 32

Fig. 33

Sitting (Figs 32–33)

Fig. 32   It will be a long time before he is able to sit without help, as his uncontrolled movements throw him off balance.

Fig. 33   When he is sitting he needs support where it will help him find his centre of gravity, this gives him stability.

Mobility is the most obvious, although not necessarily the most important, and is the activity which is impaired to some extent in all children who have cerebral palsy. By the age of five years all ataxic children, 92 per cent of those with spastic hemiplegia, 76 per cent with spastic diplegia, 46 per cent of those with athetosis and 30 per cent with spastic tetraplegia were able to walk alone (from a small unpublished series of children born between 1955–1975).

Manipulation may be very severely affected in children who show involvement of all four limbs, and where intelligence is unimpaired electronic aids may be needed for written

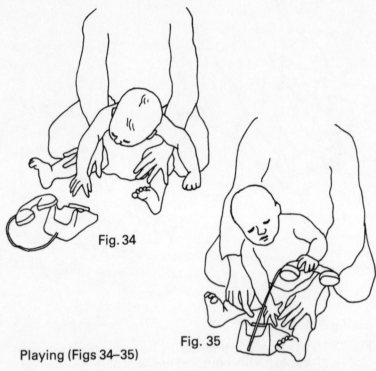

Fig. 34

Fig. 35

Playing (Figs 34–35)

Fig. 34   With this stability, his hands are freed and he is able
to move his body weight to reach for a toy.

Fig. 35   Still controlled in a stable position, he sits upright
and manipulates the toy with his hands.

work and gadgets for household activities. It is only slightly
impaired in diplegia, and hemiplegic children usually
become adept in using the affected arm as a support.
Speech is usually unaffected in hemiplegia and diplegia.
Children who have problems in all four limbs whether
spastic, ataxic or athetoid frequently manifest disorders of
expressive speech (dysarthria) typical of cerebral palsy and
athetoid children in particular may need electronic means
of communication.
Eye movements may be affected in any group of children who
have cerebral palsy.

Difficulties with *chewing*, *swallowing* and sometimes *breathing* may be encountered in the more severely affected children, and in some an early manifestation may be a difficulty in *sucking*.

Although all children who have cerebral palsy have permanent movement difficulties of some kind as described, these may be mild and cause only a minor disability or they may be sufficiently severe to cause a handicap (see p. 43).

2. Other Problems

Normal patterns

Motor development has been described in some depth, as disturbance of it is inevitable in all children who have cerebral palsy. However, a child's full development relies upon many other facets which may or may not be affected in cerebral palsy. These need to be considered, although in less detail than their motor counterparts.

Emphasis, so far, has been laid upon the intrinsic maturational basis of development of movement, which occurs in response to the environment and which enables the child to explore it and make use of it.

However, this cannot be done without the contributions of other skills and abilities, which are maturing at the same time, and being developed in response to external stimuli.

At birth the baby is only just beginning to use his vision but by one or two years of age it is normally as good as an adult's. During this time he learns first to identify objects, and then gradually to explore their size, weight and texture by the use of his improving tactile sense; to estimate distance (within limits) and follow moving objects; to see small objects and when he has developed a pincer grip to pick them up; and all this time he is assigning meaning and emotions towards everything and developing a social sense.

Hearing is very acute at birth, as the baby has been subjected to a variety of sounds, but now he needs not only to react to them but give them meaning. He appreciates and differentiates his parents' voices, and identifies everyday noises such as opening doors and food preparation. But words only start to have significance at about one year of age, and he always has to rely upon an adequate input to improve his vocabulary.

The faculties of perception, cognition, comprehension, concept formation, expression and abstract reasoning develop gradually and all depend upon an intact brain mechanism to interpret stimuli provided by an environment rich in experience.

Cerebral Palsy and its Relation to Other Skills

Vision   Sight provides one of the motivations for movement. Even in the absence of any motor difficulty children with severe visual problems show delay in the development of mobility in particular, but also manipulation and speech, so that a combination of the two disabilities has a very profound effect upon the child's development, and poses great problems for those offering help.

Hearing   A deficit in this field does not necessarily interfere with the development of movement, but may greatly delay the understanding and production of speech, which is very important for personal interaction in cerebral palsy.

Learning Difficulties   These are of three kinds: a) In many children with cerebral palsy limitations are merely motor dependent. Their 'special needs' in educational terms are only concerned with mobility and sometimes with manipulation and speech. Their understanding and ability to learn are normal and they may be of high intelligence whether their motor handicap is mild, moderate or severe; b) Another group of children, often those with minor motor impairment including spastic hemiplegia or diplegia, have 'specific learning difficulties' which do not affect their intelligence, but cause problems in formal learning, particularly of the 3Rs. This is often associated with difficulties in spatial perception or visuomotor co-ordination (Abercrombie, 1964; Wedell, 1973); c) Mental handicap. This is due to severe cerebral dysfunction; it is often but not invariably associated with severe movement disorders and in those children it may be difficult to quantify. This particular multiple handicap is one which produces the greatest problems in management and in need for support.

Social Adaptation   These are possibly the most important skills that children who have cerebral palsy need to acquire. The ability to do so rests not only upon the motor handicap, but upon the child's personality and determination, the presence or absence of other physical problems and even more upon the degree of independence and self help skills that his family and professionals are able to inculcate.

Although many children who have cerebral palsy have no other problems, in those who have, the problems react upon one another by multiplication rather than summation.

Thus a minor impairment which would not trouble an ordinary child may have a much greater effect upon the development and progress of a child who has cerebral palsy. And may be the cause of a disability becoming a handicap.

In conclusion we are considering and describing children with very diverse abilities and needs. Their individual futures depend upon how each one can cope with his compound physical problems, how he adjusts his emotional reactions to his circumstances and how he can relate to other people and develop normal social skills. The attitudes of the people nearest to him, his parents, siblings and professional contacts will have a profound effect, and the environment at home, school and in the community will contribute a great deal either positive or negative. Although his brain dysfunction is a permanent impairment which will always affect him in some way, this may be limited to disability affecting his performance in some fields, without interfering with his way of life, or it may constitute a handicap in that the child cannot fulfil a role that would be normal in his circumstances. It is the objective of parents and professionals to prevent the child's disability from becoming a handicap or, if this is not possible, to alleviate its effects.

This short description of some of the difficulties experienced by children who have cerebral palsy may be sufficient to help the reader to understand something of the complexity and diversity of problems encountered. It may serve to explain why there is no such person as a typical child with cerebral palsy, and why it is impossible to be dogmatic about any single method of treatment or education, or to limit the ways in which help may be provided. These will be discussed in subsequent chapters in Part 2.

References

ABERCROMBIE, M. L. J. (1964). *Perceptual and Visuomotor Disorders in Cerebral Palsy*. London: Heinemann Medical Books.

BOWER, T. G. R. (1977). *A Primer of Infant Development*. San Francisco: W. H. Freeman & Company.

LEVITT, S. (1984). 'Child development and the therapist' in *Paediatric Developmental Therapy*, pp. 1–12. LEVITT, S. (ed). Oxford: Blackwell.

LEVITT, S. (1984). 'Motor development' in *Paediatric Developmental Therapy*, pp. 13–33. LEVITT, S. (ed). Oxford: Blackwell.

ROBSON, P. (1970). 'Shuffling, hitching, scooting or sliding: some observations in 30 otherwise normal children', *Developmental Medicine and Child Neurology*, **12**, 608.

WEDELL, K. (1973). *Learning and Perceptuo-Motor Disabilities in Children*. London, New York and Sydney: Wiley.

3   The Family

No man is an *Island*, entire of itself.

John Donne

In the previous chapters we considered the individual children and their problems, trying to keep in mind always that it is the child as a person who matters, and not just the child with a physical difficulty. But he does not grow up in a vacuum. He is part of a family, the family is part of a wider community and all are involved in encouraging his development. The community should have much to offer, and its role will be considered more fully in subsequent chapters. It is the family members, however, who have to undertake most of the caring in a situation which is usually unexpected and invariably unique to them. They have no previous experience and very few guidelines, particularly when the child is the first in the family. A new baby always affects the parents' way of life and enforces a style of living very different from their previous existence; a baby or young child who has physical problems presents an even greater challenge.

The young child who has cerebral palsy, living as the centre of his world, may not at first be consciously affected by the anxieties and confusions that he has engendered. He has only known his own existence and until he gets about and meets peers who have greater freedom of movement, he may not realise that he is any different from other children. How he will cope with his difficulties when he realises them will very much depend upon the reactions of those around him. So that acceptance of him as he is, and a readiness to encourage independence and personal development, will be important factors in his progress.

At the outset it is the parents who have the hardest time in having to adjust to the realisation that their child has problems which they never envisaged. Ordinary children rarely turn out to be the model which their parents had in mind, but as the child grows up they grow to accept this real child who is not exactly what they expected. When a child is even more different from their anticipation this acceptance is more difficult and may be painful. The stresses encountered are usually both emotional and practical; the emotional factors are common to the parents of all children with any type of disability, but additional practical problems are encountered in many children who have cerebral palsy.

A Emotional Factors

The feelings that parents experience in these circumstances are somewhat akin to bereavement, suffering the loss of the 'perfect' normal baby whose arrival they have been anticipating with such joy.

Disbelief and *shock* at first produce numbness. Bad news of any kind seems to stun the hearer, and it may be some days before the mother and father are able to begin to take it in. All parents who have this experience prefer to be told the truth, as far as it is known, as soon as possible, but it is often necessary to have several interviews, with questions and explanations, before parents are able to consider even the barest outline of the condition of the baby or child. The presentation of the facts may be particularly difficult in cases where the baby has been premature or very ill after birth, because at the time it may not be possible to decide whether permanent brain impairment has occurred, or whether the baby can be expected to make a full recovery. The same difficulties may arise in older children who have suffered brain injury from accident or infections. This period of uncertainty is very hard, and families need a great deal of support and encouragement from all with whom they are in contact. Over-optimism is never justified, but there should always be hope. Sometimes the thought is so painful that parents take refuge in *denial*, and may be backed up by relatives and friends, refusing to admit that anything can be wrong.

Anger which may be directed at the world in general, at the professionals or inwardly upon the self leading to feelings of guilt, is a very human response. It must be accepted by the persons to whom it is directed, but where it results in guilt, reassurance must be offered time and again.

Guilt is not invariable, but sometimes is present without being expressed. It may be shown by self-doubt or self-recrimination, usually totally unfounded, resulting from events in the distant past or more recent. These need to be talked through, understood and discarded to build up the self-confidence that will be vitally necessary for helping the child with his problems.

Grief is another, almost inevitable reaction, and may show itself in a number of ways. Bursts of crying, tears at the mention of or the sight of the child, compulsion to talk about the pregnancy, the labour, the oddities of 'Uncle Jim', anything to avoid discussion of the real problem. A listening ear and a comforting presence are necessary at this time; those who want to help, relative, friend, neighbour or professional need to come to terms with the problem themselves for their support to be effectual.

However, though distressing, this stage is the beginning of facing the reality of the likelihood of the child being disabled, and may be followed by *withdrawal* (extreme inactivity) or *overactivity*.

Withdrawal may lead to loss of interest in the child, or the other children, in housework, in the spouse, or other activities in which the parent(s) previously engaged. On the other hand, *overactivity* due to the understandable longing for a 'cure' may lead to a desire to try all sorts of 'treatment' recommended by relatives, friends or neighbours, which may have the same effect of neglecting husband, home or other children.

Finally there comes a positive acceptance of the reality of the child's difficulties and a preparedness to look at the future so that, together with the professionals, a planned programme can be devised to help the child's progress and development. The time taken to work through negative feelings varies considerably, but not until this has been achieved can progress be expected. Help and counselling from a limited number (preferably one) of suitable professionals must be available during this period; hope and realistic expectation of the rate of progress should be expressed whenever possible.

B   Additional Practical Factors
The feelings and emotions described arise in the parents as a natural consequence of any disaster affecting their child, but in children who have cerebral palsy additional strains may arise from physical factors.

Intensive care whether of baby or child may necessitate separation and the almost impossibility of adequate cuddling necessary for child and parent. Moreover, early bonding between mother and newborn is inhibited or delayed.

Difficulties in handling above and beyond the physical problems of limited or abnormal movement may include *convulsions, crying* and *restlessness,* and may lead to disturbed nights for the parents and exhaustion during the day. *Feeding difficulties* may be the cause of prolonged feeding times and give less time for housework; the child may need help with feeding for a much longer period. *Dressing and undressing* are often difficult and the child may be very delayed in undertaking these tasks for himself.

Time spent on visits to hospitals may be a further factor, in expense, use of time, and physical exhaustion. The importance of close co-operation between hospital and community staff is essential to ensure reasonable demands upon the parents. Many children who have cerebral palsy learn to walk between the ages of one-and-a-half to five years so that, as they are able to feed and dress themselves, they do not pose a physical problem for their parents. However, those children who are unable to walk become more *difficult to transport* as they grow bigger and heavier, and require very much more attendance from their parents. This is also true of *children who have additional problems,* particularly visual, mental or epilepsy.

In some families, therefore, the physical burden decreases as the child grows older, in others it can be expected to increase. Hopefully the services available locally should increase with the need, and should certainly be strongly in evidence during the school years.

As children grow into their teens they experience the same teenage doubts and anxieties about the future as their able-bodied peers, only frequently these are neither noticed nor acknowledged. This may be an additional time of stress for the family and will be discussed more fully in Chapters 7 and 8.

C Siblings

Life for siblings of a handicapped child is never easy. The effect on their life style is as deep and fundamental as that on their parents, but it very often goes unacknowledged. While the parents are coping with their own range of feelings, with the practical problems of caring for the disabled child and with their physical exhaustion, it is only too easy to disregard the problems that siblings suffer. It is particularly difficult when the affected child is the second in a family, as, in addition to supplanting the first in his special role as 'our child', this new arrival is receiving an inordinate amount of attention from parents who themselves are anxious and distressed.

Simeonsson and McHale (1981) in studying the responses of siblings have found a great variety of reactions. They point out that the relationship between the affected child and siblings may be positive in many respects; the disabled child has companionship with the example of someone nearer his own age and size, and the sibling may acquire maturity and responsibility. However, if the sibling feels neglected or overburdened with physical cares, the effect on him will be entirely negative and will be reflected in the attitudes of the child who has cerebral palsy. The sibling may also feel guilt at antagonistic emotions towards his rival, or may even wonder whether something is wrong with himself. Other factors may be implicated: birth order, family size and religious convictions may all have an effect on the ability of the family to cope emotionally or practically, and in needy families the sheer physical and financial burden of extra care, and the lack of an extended family, may be too much for all to bear. The most powerful influence is that of parental attitudes. When parents have been able to understand and accept the problems they have, and are able to discuss with one another and their other children, then the whole family, supported by their chosen professionals, will be able to offer their disabled member and his siblings the greatest opportunities for development and progress.

D Crisis Periods

All families have crises, but when one member has an additional problem coping is more difficult. Such incidents as moving to a new location for a new job; illness of one or other member of the family; the arrival of a new baby; starting or changing or leaving school; death of a grandparent or other relative; or break up of the marriage, happen in all families. Ability to adjust must be based on relationships which have been established before crises occur. Therefore it is particularly important that the disabled child, during his ordinary daily life, should be able to look to others besides Mum for care and help so that when a crisis occurs, both of them will have other sources of support.

E Communication

(i) *Between parents.* This is the most obvious, most important and sometimes the most difficult. Marriages differ so much, that whereas many couples discuss absolutely everything, others find it difficult to express their feelings in words. When both are feeling bruised and uncertain, and particularly if their stages of grieving are different, verbal communication may be beyond them. A solution to this problem may be discussion together with a third person, relation, friend or professional.

(ii) *Between parents and children.* Difficulties in this situation are often a spin off from communication problems between Mum and Dad. All parents have to deal with questions about sex, illness, death and Providence from their young children, and the way they are able to deal with these will colour their ability to explain why one member of the family is different from his peers.

(iii) *Between parents and professionals.* This is perhaps the nub of the problem, and the onus is upon professionals to see that it is properly tackled. There are probably two levels of communication needed a) the communication of technical information which will usually be undertaken by the paediatrician or a member of the medical team. This will need to be a continuing process and should include: discussion of the cause of the condition once it is known; genetic advice as to the likelihood of recurrence or ways of preventing it; explanation of the help that will be needed and how it will be provided; forecast, within limits, of progress and outcome. b) A friendly relationship with a compatible member of the team who will find time for listening, further explanation and expansion of the technical information proffered, and will become a sympathetic confidante and consoler.

F Other Sources of Support
At the outset many parents will feel the need to limit their contacts, to confine their problems to their home environment and to accept a limited amount of help within it. This attitude should be respected so long as professional contact is maintained and the appropriate sources of help available and utilised.

However, the parents themselves, Mum in particular, will soon find the need to explore a wider environment, and hopefully they will find this in the local Child Development Centre, where they can meet not only professional helpers but other parents with similar problems. Details of the support available will vary according to the locality. In later chapters the types of support needed will be outlined, and sources will be described in more detail. Nationally the Spastics Society (p. 160) offers advice at its London centre, organises a number of special units and can put parents in touch with local groups.

Summary

In a careful study, Tarran (1981) suggests four requirements for a flexible and comprehensive service as a result of views expressed by families involved in the care of children with cerebral palsy:

1.   Early and continuing information about the diagnosis and its prognosis.

2.   Practical assistance with daily management problems according to the needs of an individual family, and provided at home or in some sort of day placement.

3.   A home visitor who can give assistance with the practical and emotional problems of the family.

4.   Facilities to encourage contact between parents of handicapped children, especially for mutual support.

Finally it is essential that the relationship between the parents and professionals should be built up into a partnership (Grantham and Russell, 1985). Their common aim, to help the child to achieve this potential, brings them together in the first place, then they need to develop trust in one another and to boost each other's confidence in the skills which they are able to share. How this can be done will be considered in the following chapters.

References

GRANTHAM, E. and RUSSELL, P. (1985). 'Parents as partners', in *Working Together with Handicapped Children*, pp. 38–59. Griffiths, M. and Russell, P. (eds). London: Souvenir Press.

SIMEONSSON, R. J. and McHALE, S. M. (1981). 'Review: research on handicapped children: sibling relationships'. *Child: care, health and development*, 7, 153–171.

TARRAN, E. C. (1981). 'Parents' views of medical and social work services for families with young cerebral-palsied children.' *Developmental Medicine and Child Neurology*, **23**, 173–182.

Part Two

WHAT CAN WE DO TO HELP?

4   Early Intervention

Give me a child for the first seven years and you may do what
you like with him afterwards.

A Jesuit saying

Intervention implies a 'stepping in' in order to modify action
and is very aptly applied to the additional help which needs
to be offered to any child who is delayed in development. It
is of particular importance for children who have cerebral
palsy, and those who are at risk.

Although most of the children will need some additional
help throughout their lives, it is stressed by all who work
with them that the early years are the most important, not
only for the prevention of wrong patterns of movement and
possibly even deformity, but also for the inculcation of
attitudes and relationships to encourage determination and
independence which are so important in later life.

Early in this context is taken as referring to the pre-school
years up to age five, with particular emphasis on the
first two years during which all the basic developmental
functions are attained.

In searching for a flexible and comprehensive service
suitable for all children who have cerebral palsy it is
appropriate to consider the requirements put forward by
parents as described by Tarran (1981) (see Chapter 3,
p. 52).

1.   Early and continuing information about the diagnosis and its prognosis

Whenever and however consideration is given to helping
children and their families, this always has to be a team
project; no one person can ever expect to have all the skills
necessary. At the same time no child or his parents wish to
be confronted by a bevy of earnest strangers anxious to do
their bit. Great care has to be taken by the team to ensure
that the most suitable spokesperson be selected for each
family.

Information is a two way process, so the relationship between giver and recipient needs to be open and trusting. The way in which information is offered is as important as its content; there should always be plenty of time for question and answer; the informer must be prepared both to listen and to understand the unspoken queries that lurk behind the verbal conversation (Freeman and Pearson, 1978). There may need to be two levels of professionalism involved: one the technical specialist who may need authority and experience e.g. a paediatrician; the other a member of staff with more time and a less threatening persona, often able to communicate more easily with the parents. It must always be appreciated that information given can never be wholly absorbed nor understood in conditions of emotional stress, and that the initial interviews must be followed up soon and frequently. Even during early childhood there will be changes in the needs of any child as he develops and makes progress. It is important that the continuing information is consistent, which makes it essential that the team should be closely knit and co-operative. Wherever possible information should be allied to action, and should always contain elements of encouragement and hope, always pointing out even the slightest gains and emphasising all signs of improvement.

Early information should perhaps be defined as immediate, and will need to be presented under different circumstances:

a) During the neonatal period. Some babies, particularly those nursed in intensive or special care, may give cause to suspect that there may have been some hazard to brain development. In certain units where there are advanced diagnostic facilities this may be verifiable during this period (see Chapter 11). At this point it is usually impossible to do more than warn the parents that the baby may have sustained impairment of brain function, although the outcome, whether full or partial recovery or more severe disability or even handicap, cannot be predicted. This is a difficult period for professionals and parents; there may have been fear even as to the baby's survival, and the continuing uncertainty is hard to bear. Mutual trust and confidence is essential and it is always helpful and advisable to initiate developmental advice and help, giving the parents encouragement and hope from this early stage. It is often a great support to involve the physiotherapist while the baby is still in the neonatal unit (Murphy, 1984).

b) As a result of developmental screening (Griffiths, 1973; Drillien & Drummond, 1983). In the United Kingdom facilities are available for all babies for developmental screening to be carried out by doctors or health visitors, either in local welfare clinics, health centres, GP premises or follow-up clinics in the local hospital. Those who do not or cannot attend are usually seen within their homes. Where any delay is noted, the baby may be seen again in a month or, where the delay is marked or there are suspicious signs, may be referred to the team at the Child Development Centre (see p. 74 and Chapter 5).

c) The parents themselves, or relations or friends may notice that the baby or child is not progressing as expected, and these reports must be taken seriously. When advice is sought from the health visitor or GP it is likely that, if these impressions are confirmed, referral will be made to the Child Development Centre.

d) During an acute episode in hospital, in an older child, due to illness or injury. If children experience an episode of unconsciousness of any length of time there is always a risk of some permanent impairment of brain function, and the problem of giving information is similar to that experienced in the newborn period.

Diagnosis refers to being able to say exactly what the trouble is and why. It may be weeks or sometimes months before the type and extent of the brain dysfunction becomes clear, even if the cause has been apparent for some time. It is important, wherever possible, to apply a 'label' to the condition, although this is not absolutely necessary for deciding the help that is needed, which usually depends upon function. However, the more precise definition provided by the label makes it easier for the parents to accept the child's difficulties and for the professionals to understand the child's needs.

Prognosis refers to foretelling the future for the child. In the early days, although frustrating for parents, it is necessary to be very cautious both as regards the rate of progress and the eventual outcome. These depend upon a number of factors and will be determined not only by the severity of the motor difficulty but by many extraneous conditions such as the presence of other disabilities, the child's temperament and motivation, the way he is encouraged at home and elsewhere and the standard of help that is available to him. Comprehensive and continuous assessment (see Chapter 5) will be absolutely essential to identify strengths and weaknesses, and to plan strategies to make use of the one and overcome the other. Response to the help then given is one of the most powerful indications of progress and the eventual outcome.

Continuing information   The necessity for continuing information should now be apparent—as the professional team receives new information from the results of tests that have been carried out; from the findings of the assessment procedures; and from the child's progress and response to practical measures undertaken to help him. This information will need to be relayed to the parents, and their information about the child received and integrated into reports and procedures.

2.   Practical assistance with daily management problems according to the needs of an individual family, and provided at home or in some sort of day placement

The practical assistance given to parents in the daily management of their child, is probably the most comforting contact they have, when faced with the innumerable problems of day-to-day living. Careful evaluation of their problems should be made, and the resulting advice must be acceptable to the family. Direct involvement of the parents as 'therapists' under professional guidance may increase their source of competence (Freeman and Pearson, 1978). However, this may work adversely in that if the child does not improve, the parent may begin to reject the child (Kogan et al, 1974), hence the need for correct assessment. Practical intervention should be geared towards:

1. Help with routine activities and teaching parents;
2. Prevention of deformity;
3. Aids to help daily activities;
4. Promotion of normal development and movement.

Routine activities (1)
These include such things as feeding, bathing, toileting, sleeping, dressing and playing, and during all these activities a daily programme may be built up to promote normal development.

Because correct positioning and handling is important for the development of normal posture, so much a part of daily management, the home visitor assessing the child's physical difficulties which are causing the mother's problems, will usually be a paediatric physiotherapist.

Feeding is usually the most time consuming of the daily activities, often causing stress and tension in the mother if the baby is difficult by refusing to suck. This can often be eased by finding a comfortable position for both mother and child, where the child may feel secure and so learn to relax, thus promoting better feeding. All activities should be a happy interaction between the mother and her child, but of all, perhaps feeding is the one which promotes bonding, love and acceptance. It should be a pleasurable experience and a time of the day to look forward to. Successful feeding times will encourage and produce feelings of confidence in the mother.

Bathing, toileting and dressing are all times which may be combined, by correct handling, to promoting the child's development. Ways may be found to develop head control. Close, body contact, with the child responding to the mother's movements in her handling are a secure and comforting way for the child to learn. Dressing can be done on the lap instead of on the bed. Learning to lie the child on his tummy while being dressed will help him to learn to lift his head. Potty training can be done during a quiet sit down, with the potty between the mother's knees or feet and her child supported in a good sitting position by her body or legs while watching television or reading a story. Bathing is a time when kicking may be encouraged. It is often easier if a parent gets into the bath with the child and supports him on her lap. Parents often find this out for themselves.

Playing and social interaction will be woven into all these activities. Play is the most useful learning tool of all and should be an integral part of all daily management, not thought of as a 'time to be set aside'.

Aids and prevention of deformity (2 and 3)
The number of aids available is increasing all the time and it can often be very confusing to choose which is the best thing to use at any one time. A useful guide is only use them when absolutely essential. It must not only make the home management easier, but it must also promote the child's learning and help prevent deformity.

Aids may be used as a carry over of things learnt during the daily activities. They may help potting (as the Watford Potty Chair, Finnie (1974)), lying, sitting, standing and moving. Each one can be related to helping an activity. Special seating needs careful selection, with good posture being the guiding factor. With good seating the child will use his hands better, he will follow his mother's movements with his eyes and learn head control. As he begins to gain his own balance the support should be gradually taken away.

Side lying boards will help midline, eye/hand control, and standing frames will aid skeletal formation, especially at the hips with weight bearing, together with helping constipation problems, kidney and lung function.

Walking aids such as baby trucks with a weight in for support, or ladder back chairs and special boots with or without splints, will aid independent walking. Specific aids, such as those for bathing and toileting, will often be helpful, and toys will help with learning and fine motor skills. The use of an aid needs careful monitoring and it should not be seen as a permanent fixture, only as a means to an end, and something which can be changed or discarded as the need arises.

Promotion of normal development (4)
The daily management programme is planned to help normal development through the correct continuous handling and stimulation of the child. There are many forms of treatment techniques which may be used to promote development, but as has already been stressed it is the normal everyday handling which will help the child towards his independence. Physiotherapeutic methods will be explained to the parents, with careful regard as to how this is incorporated into the day to day activities. The treatment procedures should become a way of life rather than a time to be set aside to do exercises with the child. The help given towards encouraging the child to move must be according to what he needs, and must be adapted and changed as he changes, grows and develops.

It will be seen from this that the main responsibility will rest on the physiotherapist, who will use, from her background experience, the most effective ways of promoting good movement patterns in each individual child. This may involve a neurological approach as advocated by Bobath and Bobath (1984) or a learning experience as in Conductive Education (Cotton, 1974; Seglow, 1984). Many workers manage to combine the principles of these and other approaches in their programmes for individual children.

3. A home visitor who can give assistance with practical and emotional problems of the family
The practical problems in the home may be domestic, financial or technical, related to special needs of the cerebral

palsied child. The technical problems will largely have been dealt with in Section 2 of this chapter, and indeed the home visitor may well turn out to be the physiotherapist who is advising on the management of day-to-day problems arising in the home, and very likely visiting the day centre which the child may be attending.

If the home visitor is not the physiotherapist there is still this role to be played on the technical side, in liaising with the team at the Child Development Centre (see Chapter 3), in helping the mother to carry out some of her necessary tasks, in co-operating with the toy library and contacting any local self-help groups.

On the domestic scene a large variety of problems may be encountered. In any household a small child always creates a number of problems, tussles over feeding, toileting, dressing, answering innumerable endless questions, shopping, cleaning, cooking, all comprise a very busy day finishing with bath and bed-time. These problems are exacerbated when a child has cerebral palsy, as every task takes so much longer and there are additional activities relating to the disability that need to be fitted in. A home visitor can help to organise the day's routine, can listen to and discuss all kinds of problems, may help to organise sessions at some day care centre or help to arrange baby sitting facilities, and liaise with the Family Fund (see Chapter 9) to obtain a clothes washing machine and possibly other gadgets.

With regard to finance, the visitor should be able to advise the mother about additional allowances to which she may be entitled. The Citizen's Advice Bureau can often help (see Chapters 9 and 10).

The emotional problems that are likely to beset parents of children who have cerebral palsy have been outlined in Chapter 3. It is essential that the home visitor should have a knowledge of the stages through which the parents need to pass and be able to identify their present status and needs. Other problems familiar to all families may arise which occur in ordinary households such as marital disharmony, sibling rivalry and jealousy, but which are more frequent in, and even precipitated by, the presence of a handicapped member.

Thus the home visitor faces a difficult but vital task and needs a daunting list of talents and expertise: time to spend and reliability; ability to empathise with the family, to listen and to communicate; some knowledge of the disability and its effect on the particular child; a knowledge of available resources. This is asking a great deal of any individual and it illustrates how necessary it is that the person undertaking the assignment should have the close backup of a multi-disciplinary team and be part of it. Also, it is important that the home visitor should be selected as someone who will be welcomed by the family for herself (or himself), as a person rather than for the profession represented. When it is a question of imparting knowledge this can be passed on from the team, but personal support and understanding must come from the individual.

Who, then, can undertake this kind of work? Is any professional skill necessary? If so, what? These questions are answered to some extent in Tarran's paper (1981), previously referred to. She asked the parents which professionals had been most helpful. Classed as very helpful were family doctors 50 per cent, consultant paediatrician 73 per cent, social workers and home visitors 57 per cent, health visitors 27 per cent, physiotherapists 71 per cent; unhelpful were ten per cent of family doctors, four per cent of consultant paediatricians, 11 per cent of social workers, 27 per cent of health visitors and six per cent of physiotherapists. These figures are in some contrast to those from Hewitt's (1970) findings in which 56 per cent of family doctors, 74 per cent of consultant paediatricians, 61 per cent of social workers and home visitors, 75 per cent of health visitors and 42 per cent of physiotherapists were rated as helpful. The differences probably relate to specialised training of health visitors and physiotherapists, and to local attitudes and resources. It can be postulated from these reports that it is the right person with the right training in the right place at the right time who will be the most helpful home visitor.

Of the four professions most likely to have the time, one would expect the following, noting their assets from their basic training and their needs for further experience.

Social workers are well trained in family dynamics and experienced in emotional problems, domestic difficulties and financial queries. They need the added support of the multidisciplinary team in knowledge of the way the disability affects the individual child and the practical measures necessary to help him and his family.

Home visitors may have different skills according to their own background and the way in which local services are run. For instance in the Honeylands project (Carlyle, 1980), the home visitor to a child with cerebral palsy would be a home therapist and most probably a phsyiotherapist. The Portage project (Cameron, 1982) was developed in Wisconsin, USA and has been adopted in various parts of the United Kingdom, particularly Wessex and South Glamorgan—home visitors are trained in a simple method of encouraging child development and may come from a variety of backgrounds (often health visiting). However, although the programme is highly effective for developmentally delayed children, it has been found to be less effective for children who have cerebral palsy (Barna et al, 1980; Bidder et al, 1983). If it is used for these children the home visitor should work under the supervision of a physiotherapist.

Health visitors (public health nurses) have the advantage that, by the nature of their employment, they know the family well, and may have been acquainted with the mother during her pregnancy. They are trained in child development and well acquainted with common childhood illnesses and behaviour disorders. They may be less well grounded in the clinical features of cerebral palsy but can easily be made aware of the problems in individual cases.

Paediatric physiotherapists are those who have the most to

offer in the way of practical assistance with daily management, and will almost certainly have had contact with the
family from the time the disability was diagnosed and
hopefully from the time the risk was suspected. Their
ability to cope with the emotional and personal problems
varies according to their temperament, but they should
always be deeply involved with the home visitor if he/she is
a separate person.

4. Facilities to encourage contact between parents of handicapped children, especially for mutual support

The 'special needs' of parents with a handicapped child are
as specific as those of the child they love and care for. They
need to meet other parents with similar problems; worries
should be recognised and catered for. Once help in the
home is firmly established and confidence is growing, both
mother and baby will benefit by mixing with others for
social support and professional guidance. This could be one
of the many roles of the local Child Development Centre, or
may be set up in a community based centre where the
facilities are thought to be suitable. Such therapeutic
groups may cater for children with any type of developmental delay, for example, the Armitstead Centre in Dun-
dee (Tarran, 1979); the Baby Group at Ridge Hill, Dudley
(Clegg, 1984), incorporating hydrotherapy (Plate 1), with
added professional advice from such people as the dietitian
and the community nurse (Plate 2); or a specialist group
for children with cerebral palsy set up in a quiet area of a
local hospital, using some of the principles of conductive
education (Seglow, 1984) under the guidance of the
physiotherapist (Plate 3).

The mixed units in particular will offer not only social and
professional support, but also an introduction into assessment. Groups such as these give the parents a chance to
chat among themselves, to watch the responses of other
mothers and children, to ask informally all the questions
which are worrying them, and at the same time, believing

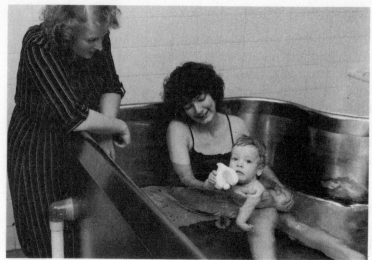

Plate 1   The mother is looking on, the physiotherapist in the pool with the child. Hydrotherapy for young children in a warm small pool has social and physical benefits and encourages the child's confidence in movement.

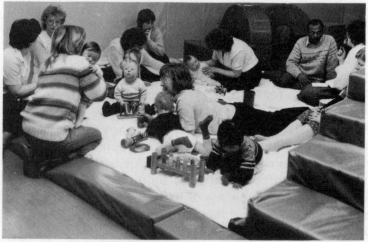

Plate 2   A group of mothers (and one father who is talking to the dietician) in a group housed in the hospital unit at Dudley. It can be seen that the children have varied disabilities (several children who have Down's syndrome can be readily identified); the two children in the foreground have cerebral palsy. The interaction between parents and with the children is clearly seen. This is an early situation in which a number of professionals can be involved on an informal basis.

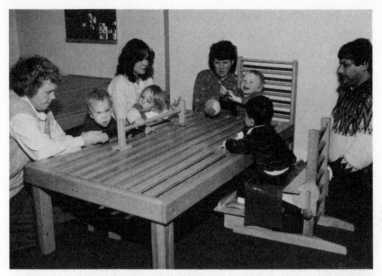

Plate 3   A more advanced pre-school parent and child
group working together, based on Conductive
Education principles.

the best ways to help their own child, and boost their
confidence (Plate 2).

In these units all the children attending have problems
which need professional guidance, but there is also a need
for mother and child to start to mix with ordinary children.
In some situations an 'opportunity class' associated with
Pre-School Playgroup Association may be available, in
which the clientele is 50 per cent 'ordinary' and 50 per cent
children with neurodevelopmental problems. Here there is
a very high representation of mothers and less professional
input. More often a place may be found in an ordinary
playgroup with fewer mothers helping with a prepon-
derance of ordinary children. The Pre-School Playgroups
Association booklet offers excellent advice to playgroup
supervisors on how to accommodate and help children
with any kind of developmental problem. Amongst their
recommendations are that handicapped children should be

limited to about one in ten, that parents should be con-
sulted and given full explanations, and that close contact
should be maintained with the professionals involved.
Whichever way of mixing with ordinary children is chosen,
it serves as an introduction to nursery education, and gives
a guide to the child's needs for integration into mainstream
schooling. As well as these there may be a 'drop-in' group
one afternoon a week where parents are welcome to come
to the centre, meet, have tea, chat or perhaps have a talk
about other subjects.

Whilst maintaining a relationship with the professionals
the parents may wish to meet quite independently and
arrange their own agenda. One such group started in the
West Midlands with the support of the Spastics Society.
This support encourages fund raising events to raise money
for various functions. This group is called PIN, 'Parents in
Need', and although professionals are welcome and often
invited, it is felt that it should be just for parents, with the
advice and help coming from the 'Parent Group' when
needed.

A more formal group may be arranged by the local
Portage Team to discuss specific points arising from their
input into families (Cameron, 1982).

There are many other special groups, often set up for
those who have an interest in one particular handicap.
These are only useful if there are sufficient in number in the
local area. Sometimes regional organisations run groups of
specific interest, although this becomes a much more
formal occasion.

It is usual that there is a need for both formal groups,
where parents feel they learn more about their problems,
and informal groups where not only the parents can learn
but the professionals may learn more about the needs of the
parents. Whatever is offered the meetings should be seen
as a partnership with the professional group, thus creating
an equal relationship.

References

BARNA, S., BIDDER, R. T., GRAY, O. P., CLEMENTS, J. and GARDNER, S. (1980). 'The progress of developmentally delayed pre-school children in a home training scheme', *Child: care, health and development*, **6**, 157–164.

BIDDER, R. T., HEWITT, K. E. and GRAY, O. P. (1983). 'Evaluation of teaching methods in a home-based training scheme for developmentally delayed pre-school children', *Child: care, health and development*, **9**, 1–12.

BOBATH, K. and BOBATH, B. (1984). 'The neurodevelopmental treatment' in *Management of the Motor Disorders in Children with Cerebral Palsy*, pp. 6–18. SCRUTTON, D. (ed). Spastics International Medical Publications; Oxford: Blackwell; Philadelphia: Lippincott.

CAMERON, R. J. (ed). (1982). *Working Together—Portage in the U.K.* Windsor: NFER/Nelson.

CARLYLE, J. (1980). 'A paediatric home therapy programme for developmental progress in severely handicapped infants', *Child: care, health and development*, **6**, 339–350.

CLEGG, M. (1984). 'Mother and baby groups', *Therapy*.

COTTON, E. (1974). 'Integration of treatment and education in cerebral palsy', in *The Handicapped Person in the Community*, pp. 217–221, BOSWELL, D. M. and WINGROVE, J. M. London: Tavistock Publications and Open University.

DRILLIEN, C. and DRUMMOND, M. (1983). *Developmental Screening and the Child with Special Needs*. London: Heinemann; Philadelphia: Lippincott.

FINNIE, N. R. (1974). *Handling the Young Cerebral Palsied Child at Home*. London: Heinemann.

FREEMAN, R. D. and PEARSON, P. H. (1978). 'Counselling with parents', in *Care of the Handicapped Child*, pp. 35–47. APLEY, J. (ed). Spastics International Medical Publications; London: William Heinemann Medical Books; Philadelphia: Lippincott.

GRIFFITHS, M. I. (1973). 'Early detection by developmental screening', in *The Young Retarded Child*, pp. 11–19. GRIFFITHS, M. (ed). Edinburgh and London: Churchill Livingstone.

HEWITT, S. (1970). *The Family and the Handicapped Child*. London: Allen and Unwin.

KOGAN, K. L., TYLER, N., and TURNER, P. (1974). 'The process of interpersonal adaptation between mothers and their cerebral palsied children', *Developmental Medicine and Child Neurology*, **16**, 518–527.

MURPHY, F. (1984). 'The physiotherapist in the neonatal unit', in *Paediatric Developmental Therapy*, pp. 63–75. LEVITT, S. (ed). Oxford: Blackwell.

PRE-SCHOOL PLAYGROUPS ASSOCIATION. *Guidelines for Playgroups with a Handicapped Child*. London: Pre-school Playgroups Association (see Chapter 10).

SEGLOW, D. (1984). 'A Pattern of Early Intervention', in *Paediatric Developmental Therapy*, pp. 76–87. LEVITT, S. (ed). Oxford: Blackwell.

TARRAN, E. (1979). 'Armitstead mother's group—a support group for mothers of young handicapped children', *Social Work Today*, **4**, p. 16.

TARRAN, E. C. (1981). 'Parents' views of medical and social work services for families with young cerebral-palsied children', *Developmental Medicine and Child Neurology*, **23**, pp. 173–182.

5 Assessment

From each according to his ability to each according to his need.
Karl Marx

The term 'assessment' calls up a number of images and very often has a frightening impact upon parents who may at first look upon it as a grim kind of pass or fail examination. This impression is far from accurate and, using Kipling's 'honest serving men' quoted in Chapter 1, it is helpful to answer many of these unspoken questions in this way. Before doing so, however, generalisations are important. First, assessment can never depend upon a single interview, and second, it can never be effectively carried out by a single person, however experienced; it must be continuous and comprehensive. Individual members of a team need to use their expertise in their specialist activities and together continue to observe the child's progress in all fields in response to the help that is being given.

WHAT is assessment?
In this context it is a continuing evaluation of a child's attainments in all fields of development, based on a detailed estimation of his abilities and disabilities. Hence, it is very different from an examination which only takes account of attainment. The team not only looks at how the child is performing in relation to his chronological age, but also analyses what he can do and where he is failing. Using this knowledge strategies can be worked out to help to counteract his disabilities and encourage his abilities. The parents are always asked to take part. As the child progresses changes can be made to the tasks he and his parents are given and help from the professionals is adjusted accordingly.

Careful records are kept by all members of the team, who work in close collaboration with one another and with the parents, always trying to ensure that only one of their number is the 'key worker' in direct contact with the family, but liaising closely with other members of the team who are involved.

WHY is it necessary?

1.   The first aim is to define as accurately as possible all fields of development in which the child shows delay or difficulty, at the same time noting where he is able to function at a level one would expect for his chronological age.

2.   Having defined those areas in which he is lacking ability and those in which he is able, it then becomes possible for the professionals to offer the kind of help that he needs. The programme for each child will need to be carefully tailored according to his profile of attainments at the time, will be planned with the approval of the parents and all members of the team, and will be carefully monitored to adapt to changes in progress and attainment.

3.   Full reports from the assessment records can then be used as the child is coming up to school age to prepare the 'statement' which will help to decide the most suitable school placement, and to alert the authorities at the chosen school of the difficulties that a child may have which constitute his 'special educational need'.

WHEN should it be carried out?

There is no one time for a procedure which is intended to be continuous, nor is there any schedule which states at what times or in what order specific skills should be evaluated. Formal assessment can rarely be carried out in children under two years of age, and advice has to be offered on an *ad hoc* basis usually beginning with help towards movement undertaken by the physiotherapist. As she observes and encourages movement, correcting it where necessary and showing the mother how to handle the baby, she will be able to deduce the type and extent of the motor impairment and an experienced therapist will be able to notice delay or deviance in other fields of development. Indeed, these may have already been highlighted during the routine developmental screening described in Chapter 4 (p. 57).

Parents may ask for education for their children with special needs from the age of two years and if they do so, formal assessment will be necessary. However, if the facilities provided by the health service and social services are adequate, the parents may feel that playgroup placement may be all that is needed at that time. The placement of pre-school children in playgroups and nursery units has been discussed in Chapter 4 and the decision will largely rest upon the parents' desires and the availability of local resources.

Before formal school entry at the age of four to five years, any child who is expected to have 'special educational needs' will be provided with a statement, compiled by professionals who know him, from the health authority, the local education authority (including psychologists) and the parents. This should provide a profile of the child which will help the local education authority to offer a place at the school most suited to his needs. In order for the statement to be compiled, suggestions to be made about a suitable school and consultations to take place between the head of the school, the parents and any professionals who can offer information and advice, the information will need to be collated before four-and-a-half years of age and the assessment process will need to commence when the child is two-and-a-half to three years of age.

Once a child has a statement, a review at the age of twelve-and-a-half is mandatory although assessment, both formal and informal, will continue throughout his school life, and annual review is usually very helpful.

Perhaps the most important time is prior to leaving school. The educational assessment of some able, lightly handicapped children of an academic bent can consist of the ordinary public examinations, sometimes with special allowance for physical difficulties which slow them down. For most children who have cerebral palsy assessment for post-school needs will take more note of physical capabilities, communication and social skills, ability to mix and to form relationships, and temperament and personality.

Here again, the assessment needs to be completed well
beforehand to give time for establishing the needs and
abilities of the young person and for discovering a suitable
placement.

WHERE is it carried out?
The main need is for it to be a place where the child can feel
really at home and be responsive, hence taking the child to
a strange place for a series of unexpected 'tests' can never
give a true picture of what the child is able to accomplish.
Moreover, the aim at first is to find out what sort of needs
there are both for helping the child and the carers, so that
although home is not the right place for a formal assessment, it is the right place to start. The home visitor or key
worker needs to evaluate the physical facilities and the
quality of relationships within the family, to note how the
child fits in and how the environment supports him. With
this background the physiotherapist (who may or may not
be the home visitor) can assess the degree to which the
family will be able to help her to facilitate and improve the
child's motor skills, and to encourage progress in all fields
of development.

As the mother's confidence grows and the infant becomes more able to interact with strangers, they can be
introduced to a mother and toddler group. As the surroundings become familiar and friendly to the child he will
tolerate contact with other members of the team, and in the
play situation will soon co-operate in tests of vision and
hearing, and take part in play activities which will widen
his fields of communication and social skills.

Next in a play group situation, either in the local Child
Development Centre or a nursery unit 'early learning' can
take place under the guidance of trained staff, nursery
nurses or nursery teachers, working to programmes devised by the therapists in the team and looking forward to
the time when a formal assessment report will be expected,
and will eventually become the core information in the
'statement'.

School is a place for continuous assessment for all children, and if it has been rightly selected should be a place where the child has been happy and successful, able to fulfil his potential, however limited. It is particularly important during school life that assessment and expectation should be realistic, so that in the difficult transition to adulthood on leaving school the final assessment may lead to suggestions for jobs, further training, or special care that are possible and practical and right for the individual.

HOW is it carried out?

The key word is comprehensive. It is only too easy to concentrate upon the major difficulty. In children who have cerebral palsy a motor disability is invariably present, and because this is always obvious it is likely, often rightly, to attract the most attention. So that in setting up assessment procedure, it is essential on this occasion to adhere to a fairly rigid formula and to ensure that every aspect of development is thoroughly monitored.

Evaluation of Motor Competence

Assessment is a prerequisite for any physical treatment (Nash, 1977) and is a continuing process of evaluating a child's competence; and in the eyes of the parents, nothing is more important than that of his motor ability. How often do we hear the words, 'Will he walk?', or 'When will he walk?' The continuous monitoring of his motor function gives us the knowledge and baseline from which to plan a realistic and non-failing future.

Because of the wide variety of resources and approaches of treatment available, a thorough ongoing assessment of his needs is essential before we can plan his treatment/ management programme. We need to know what he can do, what he cannot do, and more importantly, why he cannot do these things. The answers to these questions will give the physiotherapist the starting point for her planning. However, it must be stressed that although a more formal assessment may take place at certain times during the child's life, the overall treatment programme will be constantly changing as the child matures, develops and achieves.

Motor competence is usually divided into two broad areas: gross motor skills and fine motor skills. Before these areas can be assessed we need to look at the overall picture of the child, to find out what may be preventing him from achieving his goals. All types of cerebral palsy will fall into these headings.

1. *General observations*—what we observe, not only when we very first see the child, but on every occasion when we see him again, will help to tell us a lot about his future achievements. His interaction with the people caring for him and with his surroundings have a major impact on his achievements.

We look for his interest and his receptiveness, together with his movement responses.

2. *Posture and position*—It is necessary to note whether or not he can maintain with comfort the main positions he needs from which to perform a functional movement, lying, sitting and standing (Figs 3–15, Chapter 2). Can he control this position and then move?

3. *Primitive reflex activity*—One of the most disabling reasons for lack of movement in a child with cerebral palsy, is the persistence of the primitive reflexes. The reflexes described in Chapter 2 act to give him stereotyped, uncoordinated and uncontrollable responses as in athetosis (Figs 24 to 35, Chapter 2) whereas the normal undamaged child will perform a movement with ease (Figs 3–5, Chapter 2), as the brain matures and the primitive reflexes become suppressed. These reflexes also interfere with the development of normal postural reactions which serve to bring us to a stable upright position.

4. *Muscle Tone*—Muscle tone in the normal child will be in a state of readiness to perform or respond to a movement. Tone may increase in one group of muscles whilst relaxing

in another group, as he prepares himself in response to a stimulus. In the child with cerebral palsy, the muscle tone may be either too high (hypertonia) or too low (hypotonia). This will mean that he will find movements difficult to make (Figs 16–20, Chapter 2).

5. *Contractures and Deformities*—Limited movement within joints caused by continuous contraction of the muscles surrounding it, will severely interfere with the freedom of movement and eventually cause deformity of the joint, sometimes, particularly in the hip, to the extent of dislocation. Joints need a free range of action for normal movements to be produced. Severe contractions will lead to a permanent deformity which will restrict the child's abilities. Another consideration which may restrict movement, is the presence of pain caused by moving with that deformity present. Contractions and deformities will usually only occur in older and more severely handicapped children.

6. *Muscle Power*—This is generally not considered to be very important when assessing a child with cerebral palsy. However, in the older child, lack of movement and limitation of use lead to atrophy of muscles.

7. *Sensory Feedback*—It is important not to rule out the possibility of sensory losses in joint and skin, which impair sensations which are needed to experience sensory motor learning (White, 1984). A child with additional spatial and perceptual problems will often present as the clumsy child (Gordon and McKinlay, 1980). However, sometimes a cerebral palsied child with a more severe motor difficulty will have these associated problems, often resulting in poor co-ordination and this should be noted.

Following a careful assessment of the above points, we can then look at the movements the child can do.

Gross motor skills—This is usually assessed by the physiotherapist who looks at a progression of movement which includes head control and maintenance of a good posture in relation to gravity. Can he roll, crawl, sit, kneel and get up to standing? Is he able to step, with or without help? (See Figures 16–35 in Chapter 2.) All formal observation of such ability must be recorded from time to time as the child develops. The headings on the form may vary from unit to unit, but the end result will be the same.

Fine motor ability—This is usually the field of the occupational therapist. She will be looking at fine manipulative skills and eye/hand co-ordination. This assessment should only be done following an assessment of gross motor function, as so often failure to perform finer skills is due to poor gross motor function (Finnie, 1974).

Evaluation of Other Disabilities

Assessment is concerned with the whole child; ability or disability in any field will affect his performance and potential. When a child has cerebral palsy it is tempting to concentrate on motor difficulties and to forget or ignore other problems or assets, but his progress will be held back by other problems and assisted by his assets.

It is also important to remember that when a child has more than one disability each interacts upon the other to increase the effect of both. Having made a careful assessment of the motor disability, it should never be assumed that all limitations are due to movement difficulties or that other activities are probably normal. It is necessary to be sure of the degree of competence in these areas so that correction or due allowance may be made for them.

Visual Competence—Good vision enables a child to become aware of the world around him and motivates him to explore it by using his hands (sometimes his mouth) and by moving around. The child with cerebral palsy may be unable to do this, and therefore his experience of space, size, weight, distance and texture is limited, even if his sight is normal. If it is impaired in any way, another avenue for learning about his world is denied to him, and his motivation to undertake the difficult tasks of manipulation and mobility is undermined. Therefore it is doubly important that his vision should be assessed and wherever possible corrected.

The orthoptist on the team is the person who can help at this stage. She will look for squint, and will use suitable testing material to find out whether the child is able to see toys or pictures or shapes of the right size presented to him; she will also see whether he is able to follow a light or a small object with his eyes.

If there is evidence that he has a squint or does not seem to see as well as he should, he will be seen by the opthalmologist (Gardiner, 1982).

Squints are of two kinds: a) due to weakness of one of the muscles which move the eyeball, a movement difficulty which is part of cerebral palsy; b) due to a difficulty in fusing the image from both eyes. Squints always need to be treated as, if they persist, the sight from the squinting eye may be suppressed.

If the child is unable to see objects clearly there may be a number of causes which the ophthalmologist will investigate (Gardiner, 1982). The tests carried out by the orthoptist may be repeated and ophthalmoscopy may be carried out. This involves both looking into the eye with a small light and also shining a light into the eye from a distance (after drops have been administered) using lenses in front of the eye to obtain correction. These investigations will elucidate any conditions in the eyeball itself, some of which can be corrected by glasses; others may not be responsive to treatment and these children will have a double handicap. When the eyes appear normal and the child has impaired vision, electronic testing of brain waves may be used. Testing of the fields of vision is often carried out in children who have hemiplegia as the child may be unable to see properly on the same side as his motor disability.

It may be difficult for a child with cerebral palsy to take part in these tests because it is difficult for him to sit up straight, to keep still, or sometimes to understand what is required. Members of the team can help, but much patience is often needed on the part of the parent and the doctor.

Hearing—Although less important than sight for the development of manipulation and mobility, hearing is an important link with the environment for communication and learning. If hearing loss is unrecognised in a cerebral palsied child of limited mobility the 'label' of mental handicap may quite wrongly be applied or, on the other hand, a child with less severe motor disability may be overactive due to frustration from inability to communicate and the same mistake may be made.

There are two kinds of hearing impairment:

a)   Conductive. This is due to interference with the conduction of sound waves through the external and middle ear. A look down the ear with an auroscope will reveal wax, or a foreign body which can be removed, or an abnormality of the ear drum which will betoken an infection of the middle ear. Hearing due to middle ear disease may come and go and may not always be detectable either by looking at the ear drum or by hearing tests, which need to be repeated from time to time.. Such deafness is treatable and need not persist provided it is detected and assessed soon enough. Hearing tests are carried out to estimate whether bone or air conduction of sound is impaired, and other tests are used for the measurement of pressure in the middle ear.

b)   Sensorineural. This is due to impairment of nerve endings in the inner ear. It can be identified by the result of a battery of hearing tests which produce typical responses to pure sound. The audiometrician or audiology technician on the team works closely with the audiologist to get an accurate assessment of the hearing loss, and to go on to identify a suitable hearing aid. (More details from Yeates, 1980 or Nolan & Tucker, 1988.)

Speech—Speech is very frequently affected in children who have cerebral palsy. The normal production of speech requires a) hearing of words spoken, b) comprehension of their meaning, c) the ability to formulate and express a reply in words, and d) the ability to utter the words and phrases produced in the mind. Assessment therefore requires evaluation of all four skills. Hearing has already been considered, and tests of comprehension and expression are usually carried out at the centre by the speech therapist or psychologist (Cooper, 1984), and a favourite testing procedure is that devised by Reynell (1977).

Vocalisation and verbalisation are necessary to produce speech and each may be affected in cerebral palsy. The former needs a steady flow of air expelled from the lungs through the larynx and resounding from the palate. For this children must have good chest movements and an upright posture as well as control of larynx and palate. Once the sound has been produced it is modified by the muscles of tongue, lips and cheek to produce the consonants and vowels that make up words. The motor disability which affects speech (dysarthria) has the characteristics of the other movements in the type of cerebral palsy. Speech due to spasticity is slow and slurred and often quiet, due to low breath pressure; in athetosis it is jerky with wide variations in tone and pitch due to alterations in breath pressure; in ataxia it is monotonous and staccato.

All three therapists may need to be concerned in its assessment.

Learning difficulties—The phrase can apply to three kinds of difficulty experienced by children who have cerebral palsy:
a)   The child may have no difficulty whatever in learning from people or from the environment (including books etc), so long as information is provided in a form which can be used, and so long as the child is physically able (or assisted) to make responses, whether in practical, academic or social activities. Hence it is important that the movement difficulties have been accurately assessed;
b)   The child may have specific learning difficulties. These

problems may be encountered in ordinary children and there may be difficulties in learning to read, write, or draw, quite out of context to the child's other learning abilities. These may be described as dyslexia or clumsiness, sometimes even ascribed to laziness or dullness of intellect. The exact cause of these difficulties in normal children often cannot be defined but in cerebral palsy associations with underlying brain damage are more definite, and Abercrombie (1964) and Wedell (1973) have described visuomotor and perceptuomotor difficulties. The subject has been researched in depth and educational material has been devised for teachers, but the difficulties vary so much in individual children that each has to be assessed on its own merits by psychologist and teacher for each child (Day and Radcliffe, 1985);

c) The child may have a combination of disabilities that lead to a global pattern of learning difficulties in which he is greatly behind his peers in attainment of all skills. Whichever can be said to be the predominant handicap, the mental or the physical, the complex difficulties will pose a serious problem of management and almost invariably need special schooling. It is essential that the assessment of such children with this multiple handicap should be comprehensive and carefully carried out, that all disabilities discovered should be corrected wherever possible, and that the complexity of handicap presented would not deter the professionals and parents from keeping up the practical measures that will make life easier for the child and his carers.

Behaviour—Children who have cerebral palsy experience the same emotional difficulty as ordinary children but find it more difficult to express or control, particularly if they have any of the associated difficulties described in this chapter. In children with severe motor impairment, frustration and rebellion are more likely to be expressed as non-cooperation, disinterest or apathy, whereas in more active children where the motor disability is mild but possibly associated with limited mental capacity, hearing impairment, and/or epilepsy, overactivity and aggression are the order of the day. In these children comprehensive assessment is particularly important, as evaluation of visual or hearing impairment, difficulties of communication and learning, or epilepsy may enable specific help to be offered which, with assistance towards movement and social skills, will eliminate some of the frustrations which may precipitate the anti-social behaviour.

Epilepsy—The brain impairment in cortical lesions may be associated with scarring which can become the focus for a variety of epileptic attacks. It is a very common association in children who have spastic conditions, particularly when these are severe. Assessment of this condition implies a clinical judgement of the type of epilepsy, analysis of the electroencephalogram and careful monitoring of the anti-convulsant drug treatment.

WHO is responsible?
So far 'the team' has been mentioned several times, but not defined. It is an interdisciplinary community—based at a 'Child Development Centre' or a 'Paediatic Assessment Unit' (situated in the grounds of a hospital), or attached to a nursery school unit, or, occasionally, independent of either. Its members act severally as required for individual children, and together support each other and the family by sharing information and imparting their experience and skills in an interdisciplinary group.

Table 1 (taken from Griffiths, 1985) enumerates the members of the core team (Group A), the members specially related to the family (Group B), and specialists needed for specific handicaps (Group C). Families of children who have cerebral palsy will be involved with all the members of Groups A and B for a long period and from time to time may need the advice of any of the members of Group C.

Parents need to be involved as members of the assessment team. It may seem a daunting prospect to them to share information, opinions and feelings with a body of people each of whom has some specialist knowledge.

**Table 1.   Composition of Multidisciplinary Team
(It is assumed that parents will be an integral part
of each group.)**

GROUP A*	GROUP B*	GROUP C*
Core of professionals based at Central Unit	Professionals related to home, child and family	Specialists needed for specific handicaps
audiometrician/or audiology technician	community nurse family doctor	dentist physicians
nursery nurses	health visitor	ophthalmologist
nursery teacher	home therapist	orthopaedic surgeon
orthopist	home visitor	otorhinolaryngologist
physicians:	key worker°	psychiatrist
paediatrician	social worker	psychologists
psychologist		specialist teachers for
receptionist		hearing impaired
secretary		learning difficulties
social worker		mental handicap
therapists		physical handicap
occupational		visual handicap
physical		technical specialists
speech		audiotechnician
		optician
		orthoptist
		orthotist
		therapists
		occupational
		physical
° if not already included		speech
* in alphabetical order		

Reproduced from *Working Together with Handicapped Children* p. 34.
GRIFFITHS, M. and RUSSELL, P. (eds). (1985), with the permission of the
National Children's Bureau and Souvenir Press.

Parents have specialist knowledge, too; they are an integral
part of the child's life and important partners in the caring
process. It is only as professionals listen to parents and vice
versa that the child's real needs, which are paramount, can
be assessed, and a programme (which must be reviewed

and altered when necessary) can be planned and put into action. Some people may ask why a team should be necessary, but perhaps will agree that no individual will ever have the skill, the knowledge, the time or the strength on their own to help children with cerebral palsy. At the same time it is essential that parents should not feel overwhelmed by the number of professionals who are involved in helping their child. One member of the team who has been able to develop a positive relationship with the family should be regarded as the key worker and perform a liaison function between them and the rest of the team.

The ways in which such teams function vary considerably between different health districts and local education authorities: They work from different bases; there are differences in the composition and the skills of individual members; there may be differences in the degree of co-operation between individuals and groups; there are differences in emphasis on the importance of work with handicapped children and vast differences in the allocation of resources. It is right that some of these differences should exist, no Child Development Centre is a replica of another, and this gives opportunities for progress as we learn from one another.

With regard to the integration of disciplines, Cotton (1984) makes an interesting comparison between the multidisciplinary team, the interdisciplinary team and the transdisciplinary team contrasting them unfavourably with the 'conductor principle' which advocates leaving the management of children to one conductor. Whilst agreeing wholeheartedly with the principle of a close one to one relationship with an individual professional in addition to the parents, it seems to us essential to involve the different skills of a team in order adequately to assess a child's abilities and disabilities in specific fields. The 'key worker' (to use our description) then works directly with the child, with the back-up of a team who can offer support and advice in fields in which the 'key worker' has not the expertise nor the wider training.

Assessment should ensure that a realistic estimate can be made of a personality at the time, highlighting abilities so that strengths can be the foundation for growth and detailing weaknesses so that, as far as possible, they may be overcome. If this is understood to be a continuing process, leading to increased independence and understanding of potential difficulties, a foundation will be laid for what is bound to be a challenging future.

References

ABERCROMBIE, M. L. J. (1964). *Perceptual and Visuomotor Disorders in Cerebral Palsy*. London: Heinemann Medical Books.

COOPER, J. M. (1984). 'Speech and language development', in *Paediatric Developmental Therapy*, pp. 44–52. LEVITT, S. (ed). London: Blackwell.

COTTON, E. (1984). 'Integration of disciplines in the treatment and education of children with cerebral palsy', in *Paediatric Developmental Therapy*, pp. 246–258. LEVITT, S. (ed). Oxford: Blackwell.

DAY, R. and RADCLIFFE, M. (1985). 'Specific learning difficulties and the clumsy child', in *Working Together with Handicapped Children*, GRIFFITHS, M. and RUSSELL, P. (eds). London: Souvenir Press.

FINNIE, N. R. (1974). *Handling the Young Cerebral Palsied Child at Home*. London: Heinemann.

GARDINER, P. A. (1982). *The Development of Vision*. Lancaster: MTP Press Ltd.

GORDON, N. and McKINLAY, I. (1980). *Helping Clumsy Children*. London and Edinburgh: Churchill Livingstone.

GRIFFITHS, M. (1985). 'Assessment', in *Working Together with Handicapped Children*, pp. 27–37. GRIFFITHS, M. and RUSSELL, P. (eds). London: Souvenir Press.

NASH, M. I. (1977). 'Assessment of gross and fine motor function in cerebral palsy', in *Neurodevelopmental Problems In Early Childhood*, pp. 176–194. DRILLIEN, C. and DRUMMOND, M. (eds). Oxford: Blackwell.

NOLAN, M. and TUCKER, I. G. (1988, 2nd Edition). *The Hearing Impaired Child and the Family*, London: Souvenir Press.

REYNELL, J. (1977). *Reynell Developmental Language Scales*. Windsor: NFER.

WEDELL, K. (1973). *Learning and Perceptuo-motor Disabilities in Children*. London, New York and Sydney: Wiley.

WHITE, R. (1984). 'Sensory integration therapy for the cerebral palsied child', in *The Management of Motor Disorders in Cerebral Palsy*, pp. 86–95. SCRUTTON, D. (ed). Spastics International Medical Publications. Oxford: Blackwell; Philadelphia: Lippincott.

YEATES, S. (1980). *The Development of Hearing*. Lancaster: MTP Press.

6   Practical Measures

Success or failure does not depend on what we lack but rather upon
the use we make of what we have.

Dr E. R. Carlson*
(who was cerebral palsied)

In the previous chapter the emphasis was on finding out
the assets and abilities of young children who have cerebral
palsy so that parents and professionals can work together
to help the child to use 'what he has', and to make up for
'what he lacks'. Having defined the areas in which difficulty may be expected, ways have to be sought to enable the
child to do as much as possible for himself. Later chapters
will emphasise the importance of independence for young
people, and it is during early childhood that the foun-
dations have to be laid down for its achievement within the
range of the child's capability. Just as assessment has been
shown to be a continuing process, the practical measures
used for helping should be available throughout childhood
and, to whatever extent necessary, for the rest of that
person's life. They will not remain the same, but will
constantly change in response to the way the child or young
person begins, and continues, to 'make use of what he has'.

As a result of assessment of the child as a whole person,
his assets and disabilities in various fields have been defined, and in children who have cerebral palsy, difficulties
in movement are usually the first to be considered.

Movement Difficulties

Having assessed the child's motor competence we now
have a baseline on which to plan his treatment. So what can
we do to help with movement? There are many forms of
management available to us, some taking a neurodevelopmental approach (Bobath and Bobath, 1984), some a more
educational approach (the Peto method advocated by

*CARLSON, E. R. (1952) *Born that Way*. Arthur James.

Cotton, 1974, and Hari and Tillerman, 1984). Scrutton (1984) outlines an aim-orientated approach for individual functions for individual children with one overriding aim: 'an endeavour to guide the child towards adulthood with a purpose in life and with the best possibility of fulfilling himself.' Levitt (1984) also values the eclectic approach, and selects from different systems according to each child's problems.

All these approaches have common factors which cannot be ignored: all advocate early treatment, with the objective of the child reaching his full potential; all look at the child as a whole person (the 'holistic' approach, very well defined by the followers of Professor Peto, e.g. Cotton, 1987, Hari and Tillerman, 1984); all advocate thorough assessment as a prerequisite (e.g. Nash, 1977); motivation of the child is seen as the major form of encouragement to perform a movement.

Finally, with all approaches, team work amongst the people involved, including parents, seems to be the essential ingredient. All approaches are deemed to be suitable for all types of cerebral palsy, although a careful choice needs to be made for each individual.

The ways in which these programmes are carried out will vary. Those based on neurological development and mechanical management will require a more 'hands on' method, whereas those more educationally based will be towards the child doing things for himself and in doing so 'learning to learn' (Cotton, 1987).

The choice between 'hands on' and 'hands off' will partly depend upon the child's age (very young children are normally handled) and on his general ability. The neurodevelopmental approach is based on the acceptance that the arrest of normal motor development leads to the retention of total primitive patterns, which in turn delay the development of the normal postural reflex mechanisms needed for normal active movement.

As the child is handled in activities he receives messages from his limbs which give him the feeling of the position of

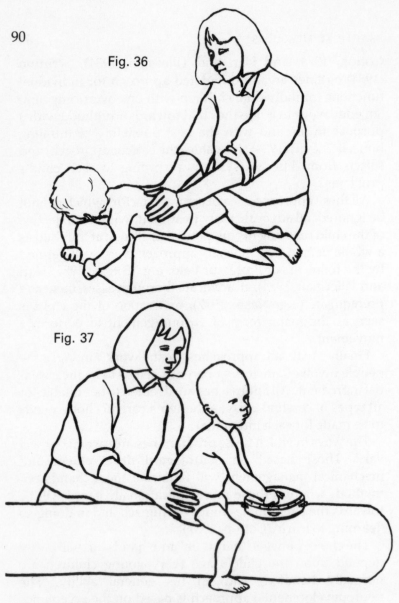

Fig. 36

Fig. 37

Fig. 36   Learning head control, with straight arms (puppy position) and forward position of the shoulders. Control and slight pressure may be given on the spine to help it to straighten and the head to lift.

Fig. 37   Sitting balance and head control on a roll which keeps the thighs separated.

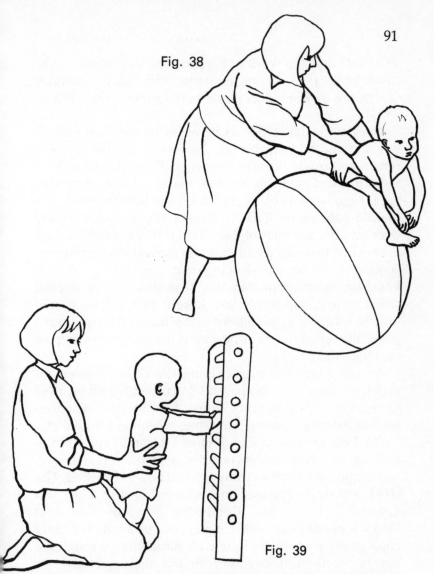

Fig. 38

Fig. 39

Fig. 38 Encouraging balance reactions and head lifting while supported and controlled with the hips at 90° or less, using a large inflatable ball as a moving base.

Fig. 39 Standing using hands for grasp. Arms are kept straight by the use of arm gaiters, which also provide sensory feedback for improving trunk control.

his joints and the work of his muscles, and so he can be guided to perform movements and adopt postures which are as normal as possible (Baddeley, 1984, White, 1984).

There is constant feedback between the therapist's handling and the child's responses, Figures 36–39. The aim is to obtain and guide his active movement of postural adjustment to handling by facilitation, making it easy or necessary for a movement to occur (Bobath and Bobath, 1984). The handling should be dynamic, never static, and should carry over into the activities of daily living. It is not essential for every child to develop and progress through the recognised sequences of normal development, i.e. rolling, sitting, kneeling, crawling to standing. It is realised that normal children do not always follow these steps and they should only be accepted as guidelines as to what might happen at a particular age. What is important is the movement pattern that the child employs.

An important factor in helping the child's movement problems is to train the parents in correct handling, thus giving the correct sensory input, for everyday activities such as bathing, toileting, dressing, washing, feeding, etc.

The Peto method or Conductive Education approach to dealing with the problems of movement in cerebral palsy is based upon the child learning to learn how to function. The child is actively engaged in his own learning (Hari and Tillerman, 1984). The Conductor educates the child through his daily activities in a group situation. The child consciously participates in what is happening through the use of 'rhythmical intention' or the singing of rhymes which denote what he is going to do next. Peto saw the problems as being mainly those of motor control, so that once a child learns to overcome his 'dysfunction' and control his motor function he becomes an 'ortho functioning' person, this being someone who could function in normal society without the use of aids or wheelchairs.

Although all parents and professionals would like to see every person who has cerebral palsy able to function completely normally in the world, it has to be acknowledged that this will not be possible for all.

The many young people (and older ones) who have cerebral palsy and are living in normal society without the use of aids or wheelchairs (illustrated by some contributors in Chapter 8) are examples of the results of their own determination, the support of their families and friends, and the effects of many different forms of treatment (or none at all).

However, even with determination, support and treatment some children who have cerebral palsy will never attain this kind of independence. As they grow, increasing weight and height make walking more difficult for some so that for these, and for those intelligent children who will never walk alone, wheelchairs give mobility, and for those who cannot talk, aids of many kinds enable them to communicate; as a result they may become independent (see Chapter 8).

Some children with multiple handicaps may never become totally independent, for these children and their carers, aids, equipment, and home adaptations will make life easier and more worthwhile (see Chapter 8).

Physiotherapists and other members of the team need in depth training and wide experience to enable them to produce, with the parents, the best programme for each child. Aids should be regarded as a way of helping the carry-over of treatment and of helping to improve the quality of life, not only for the child but also for his carers. The selection will need to be made with care. The amount of support given to the child by the aid chosen should be the minimum he needs in order to perform the function expected of him. If too much help is given then the child will cease to learn the next stage of his movement because the aid will be doing it for him. Other aids are available to help with everyday activities like bathing, washing, toileting and feeding (Finnie, 1977, Caston, 1981, Kennedy, 1984).

Plate 4 shows some examples of seating, and aids to

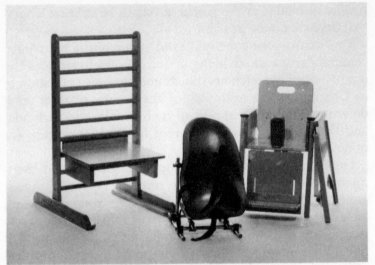

Plate 4   Seating must be carefully assessed to suit the
          needs of the child, and changed as he grows and
          improves.

walking are illustrated in Plate 5. Plates 6 and 7 illustrate a
way of helping a child to walk upstairs.

Wheelchairs, etc
Buggies, pushchairs and strollers are a useful way of trans-
porting small children. These are numerous and varied and
the choice should be considered on the parents' needs and
the best shape for the child.

Wheelchairs should only be used as a means for transport. They may be supplied with many and varied adaptations. The most important of these is a comfortable seat,
which may be firm but removable to allow folding of the
chair for taking in the car.

Children should never be left to sit for long periods in
either buggies or wheelchairs, unless a specific insert such
as a matrix or moulded seat has been supplied to help
prevent postural deformity. (For more details see Russell,
1984.)

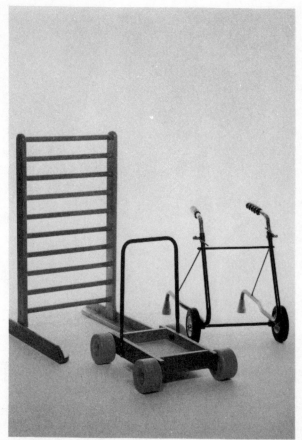

Plate 5 Some of the more common walking aids. The ladder back has dual use as a seat.

Appliances are made to the individual requirements of each child and usually take the form of splintage to help the child overcome his problems and perform his movements with greater ease and precision.

The use of appliances has greatly diminished over the years, and for a while nearly disappeared altogether. However, sometimes the use of a well assessed appliance, carefully applied, greatly enhances a child's performance.

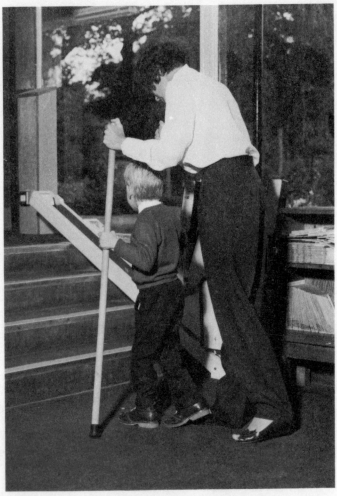

Plate 6 and 7   Helping a child to walk upstairs.

The most widely used is the Ankle Foot Orthosis or AFO.
This is a very lightweight splint, running down the back of
the leg from the knee, and incorporating the foot. The angle
at the ankle joint will help the child to keep his foot down
flat while walking, giving him better balance and stability.
These are often used in conjunction with or instead of

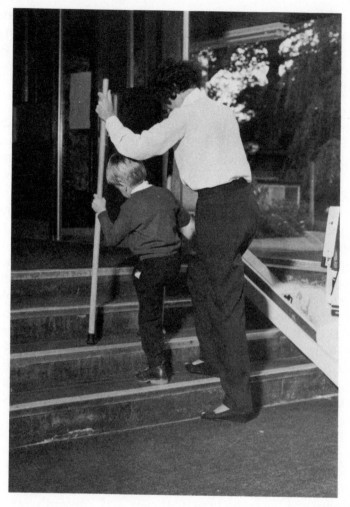

special shoes or boots, which may help to keep the feet in a good position.

Plasters may be used, particularly in spastic conditions such as hemiplegia or diplegia. Below knee plasters are applied, the foot is encased at a 90° angle for up to about six weeks. During this time the therapist will work on balance in sitting and standing, the child's active extension of his hips and knees, and perhaps the beginning of walking without much help. It has also been noted that the use of such plasters as described, giving the child more stability, will often improve hand function.

Surgery

The use of surgery in the treatment of cerebral palsy needs to be carried out in expert hands, as it can often cause more problems than it solves. It is important to remember that the success of surgery can often depend on the correct re-education of movement afterwards, and in the case of cerebral palsy this may not be possible because the damage to the central nervous system affects the child's ability to control and co-ordinate his movements. Surgery is appropriate to supplement conservative methods in some cases: in order to prevent a deformity; when pain is resulting for a deformity; to provide the child with a more stable joint. Muscles or tendons may be weakened by lengthening them but this procedure is often used to prevent a deformity from occurring, e.g. the release of certain muscles around the hip joint to prevent hip dislocation, or the lengthening of the calf muscles or the Achilles tendon at the ankle, enabling the child to put his heel to the floor and in so doing improving his stability for walking.

The age at which some operations are performed is important, as if they are done too early they may need re-doing, or if too late may be useless in preventing the deformity. The golden rule is for collaboration between orthopaedic surgeon, paediatrician and physiotherapist long before an operation appears necessary, so that sound and thorough assessment of the child's condition and progress can be made (Bleck, 1987).

Other disabilities

Visual impairment

The importance of vision to a child's development and the need for its assessment in cerebral palsied children has been mentioned already. The mutual reinforcement of two disabilities has been stressed and therefore any visual disorder must be corrected wherever possible. Glasses should be ordered if they are needed; patience and persistence on the part of the child's carers should ensure that they are worn. It may take the child a while to get used to them and to appreciate the difference they make, and special ways of fixing them may be necessary. Regular testing and where necessary change of lenses must be adhered to.

Operations for squint or cataract should be considered and arranged as in the case of other children. If these measures restore the sight to normal, then the child's education can be related to his physical difficulties alone. In some children the improvement may only bring them into the category of partial sight, which will mean that they have another special educational need and will look for very special educational help. In some children there may be no way in which their vision can be improved, and for these children early intervention needs to be exceedingly skilled. Handling is even more important when a child who has cerebral palsy is unable to see properly, and the parents need guidance from highly expert therapists and educators. The child has to learn about the world through smell, hearing and touch and because his body is unable to respond and his postural reactions are limited, he has to be helped to feel himself upright and stable, and needs extra motivation for movements (Sykanda and Levitt, 1982).

Hearing impairments
One cause of sensori-neural impairment in children who have cerebral palsy has been largely eliminated, but it still happens occasionally. The provision of hearing aids is more difficult than in other children, partly for problems of using the aid, but these should be overcome. Early intervention by trained teachers of the deaf is vital. The child's education will then depend upon his ability to master each disability, and whether he can fit into a mainstream school or will need the support of a special school for his motor or hearing difficulty.

Conductive deafness will demand the same approach as for normal children, and providing it is recognised in time, treatment should be able to restore almost normal hearing. Again, decisions about education will need to be made according to the child's overall and specific ability. (For further details see Nolan and Tucker, 1988.)

Communication
Sophisticated methods of communication are the hallmark of humanity. For children whose movement is restricted, it is important that they are also helped to communicate with others as fully as possible. To do so they need to hear (see above) and to understand what they hear. They may need extra help in this field because of their limited ability to learn of their environment, and speech therapists may help on the input side, but it is parents, other carers, and teachers who are with the child all the time who can do most. It is not easy to hold a running conversation with a child who does not ask questions, whose vocabulary is limited, and whose speech (if any) is difficult to understand, but a monologue from the adult is necessary to feed the young brain with descriptions and concepts from which to build up knowledge and understanding. In addition to the input side of communication, the child needs to express his ideas, and in many children who have cerebral palsy the mechanics of speech may be affected. In these children attention needs to be paid first of all to posture and to encouraging the child's own attempts at babbling and producing sounds before starting to mould these into words. Mueller (1974) has some very simple and practical suggestions for helping a child to start. If it becomes clear that the effort of speech is too demanding and sometimes impossible, other methods of communication will need to be used; some form of communication board (Latham, 1984), an electronic system, or, once the child can read, a language board on which his fingers or a pointer can indicate numbers, letters or common words. The DHSS has set up supraregional communication centres throughout

the country which can help and advise professionals and patients about the most suitable equipment for an individual. For written communication, when writing is difficult or impossible, adapted typewriters are the answer.

Specific learning difficulties
The child's physical condition may make some educational activities difficult, e.g. writing, handling equipment, speech, but in addition it may be found that literary or numeracy may present obstacles to learning which are quite specific. These difficulties occur in children who are intelligent and physically normal and pose a real problem to pupil and teacher which has to be assessed individually. When a child has a physical disability it is difficult to disentangle the intellectual side of the problem and to be sure whether the child has a specific difficulty or a global lack of understanding due to mental handicap. The method of teaching in these two situations has to be quite different and so it is important that the teacher, the psychologist and often the therapist should co-operate to sort it out (see p. 82).

Epilepsy
This is quite a common complication in children who have a spastic form of cerebral palsy, particularly the severe spastic tetraplegias. Clearly this adds a good deal to the problems of day-to-day management and of education, and will require drug treatment. The aim of drug treatment is to eliminate the convulsive episodes without making the child drowsy or lethargic, although this cannot always be achieved. A number of different drugs are available and often the choice is made by trial to see which is most effective in an individual case. Treatment is often long term and requires constant supervision.

General Health Care
In view of the amount of time and energy that has to be devoted to the extra care of a disabled child and the need to balance this with the general needs of the family, it is not surprising that some of the more mundane aspects of child

care may be misunderstood or neglected. So it is important that these should be considered and acted upon.

We need always to remind ourselves that a child who has cerebral palsy is, first and foremost, a child. So everything that we do for him should always be, as nearly as possible, what we would do for the ordinary child.

Diet

For the early months of life milk, and preferably breast milk, is the infant's staple food. Mixed feeding is gradually introduced after the third month, and the child becomes used to new tastes and consistencies in his food, soon developing highly personal likes and dislikes. If small changes are presented in small amounts these are more likely to be accepted. It is unnecessary to emphasise that however it is presented the food needs to comprise a well balanced diet.

In a disabled child the stages of dietary change, just as changes in mobility, manipulation and speech, may need to cover a longer period. Although the introduction of new substances and new tastes may need to be in a puréed form at first, the temptation of using this method for too long should be resisted. Very often one of the therapists may need to advise the best posture for feeding and the speech therapist may need to demonstrate how chewing can be initiated (Mueller, 1974).

All aspects of general care affect each other and it is important that diet should have a beneficial effect on other activities and aspects of care.

Sugar (including glucose) should be avoided as much as possible, particularly in sweet drinks, cakes and biscuits. This is for two reasons: 1. to prevent obesity and excessive weight gain which interfere with the child's, often limited, ability to move about; and 2. to help to avoid dental decay.

Fibre should be an essential part of the diet.

If the food intake is small for the child's age it will be wise to add vitamin supplements. These can be obtained at your local clinic or through your family doctor and it should not be necessary to pay for expensive proprietary preparations. In some units the team will include a dietitian who will be able to give advice for individual children and to fit in with ethnic and religious scruples.

Toilet Training

Most cerebral palsied children, except the very mildly handicapped, show delay in acquiring control of bladder and bowel. Fortunately it is much easier to deal with incontinence nowadays and the use of disposable nappies is the same as for the ordinary child and may continue for a longer period in a child who has cerebral palsy. If incontinence continues to be a serious problem the local health authority or social services department may supply equipment for older children, and the Family Fund may supply washing machines to needy families (Barnes, 1986).

There are, however, specific reasons why toilet training presents problems in children who have cerebral palsy:

1)   Delay in acquiring a comfortable position for lack of sitting balance. Advice from the physiotherapist or occupational therapist, and if necessary the provision of suitable equipment should remedy this;

2)   Constipation often occurs through unsuitable diet, lack of exercise and weak abdominal muscles. Advice from the team will again be necessary to find ways of counteracting this;

3)   In children who are mentally handicapped there will be delay in understanding the sensations which gradually lead a child to understand the need to respond by opening the bladder or bowel, and later to develop control and wait for a suitable opportunity. Training by reinforcement and conditioning is helpful for these children.

Sleep

All mothers and fathers are resigned to disturbed nights when they have a young baby, or when toddlers or young children are unwell. The disturbed sleep pattern may carry on from babyhood in a child who has cerebral palsy, particularly if the child is severely physically or mentally handicapped. Financial provision is offered to some extent for some children when they are older through the constant attendance allowance, but for some parents relief will only come through short periods of care for the child in a residential unit. As young children spend almost half their time sleeping, it is important for the avoidance of contractures and deformities that they should sleep in the position that is best for them. Physiotherapists and occupational therapists will offer advice in these circumstances.

Dental Care

The condition of children's teeth is extremely important for their health in childhood and in later life, and, as with other aspects, it is even more important, although more likely to be overlooked, in children who have cerebral palsy.

Measures to ensure good teeth are the same for all children: avoidance of sugary drinks (including medicines) and sticky sweet items; minimal use of dummies and banning of those that are sugar filled; regular toothbrushing; use of fluoride, this may be in the drinking water, given regularly as tablets, or applied to the teeth directly or in toothpaste.

Regular examination by a dentist is even more necessary for children who have cerebral palsy. This can be carried out in a general dental surgery or at a local health clinic. There, advice on dental hygiene, any necessary conservation treatment (filling cavities), extractions or orthodontic treatment can be carried out.

A few children may need treatment at specialist children's dentistry departments in hospital. Indications for this may be the severity of the physical handicap, making it difficult for the child to sit in a dental chair, to keep still, or to hold the mouth open adequately; or serious dental problems such as widespread dental decay, or awkward orthodontic conditions which may need specialist dental care.

Immunisation

Many infectious diseases of childhood which were previously common in the United Kingdom have almost disappeared, whilst others are much less prevalent, following the routine introduction of immunisation procedures. As with other health measures it is most important that parents of children who have cerebral palsy should make use of health facilities and ensure that their children are immunised at the appropriate times.

Some parents are concerned that there may be a risk of further 'brain damage' following immunisation, particularly if the whooping cough vaccine is involved. Certainly it seems that a very small number of children (in the region of one/100,000) may be thus affected, but the risks of death or brain damage from contracting whooping cough are infinitely greater.

The doctor responsible for immunising a child who has cerebral palsy will act upon the guidelines given by the DHSS and will probably advise that, in view of the possibility of previous brain damage, the whooping cough component should be omitted. There is no reason why the child should not be immunised against the other diseases, against which protection is now available, i.e. diphtheria, tetanus, poliomyelitis, measles, tuberculosis (in certain families) and german measles. If the child has epilepsy in any form, it is always wise to omit the whooping cough component. Your own doctor or health visitor will give advice as to the timing of the injections which can be given in the GP surgery or the local clinic.

References

BADDELEY, H. (1984). 'Motor learning'. In *Paediatric Developmental Therapy*, pp. 34–43. LEVITT, S. (ed). Oxford: Blackwell.

BARNES, E. M. (1986). *The Family Fund and how it helps.* York: Ebor Press. (Obtainable from Family Fund, P.O. Box 50, York. YO1 1UY).

BLECK, E. E. (1987). *Orthopoedic Management in Cerebral Palsy*. McKeith Press. Oxford: Blackwell; Philadelphia: Lippincott.

BOBATH, K. and BOBATH, B. (1984). 'The neurodevelopmental treatment', in *Management of the Motor Disorders in Children with Cerebral Palsy*, pp. 6–18. SCRUTTON D. (ed). Spastics International Medical Publication. Oxford: Blackwell; Philadelphia: Lippincott.

CASTON, D. (1981). *Easy to Make Aids for your Handicapped Child*. London: Souvenir Press.

COTTON, E. (1974). 'Integration of treatment and education in cerebral palsy', in *The Handicapped Person in the Community*, pp. 217–221. BOSWELL, D. M. and WINGROVE, J. M. (eds). London: Tavistock Publications and Open University.

COTTON, E. (1987) 'Conductive education'. *Association of Paediatric Chartered Physiotherapists Newsletter*, **44**, 14–17.

FINNIE, N. R. (1977). *Handling the Young Cerebral Palsied Child at Home*. London: Heinemann.

HARI, M. and TILLERMAN, T. (1984). 'Conductive education', in *Management of the Motor Disorders of Children with Cerebral Palsy*, pp. 19–35. SCRUTTON, D. (ed). Spastics International Medical Publications. Oxford: Blackwell Scientific Publications Ltd; Philadelphia: Lippincott.

KENNEDY, P. (1984). 'Aids to daily living', in *Paediatric Developmental Therapy*. LEVITT, S. (ed). Oxford: Blackwell.

LATHAM, C. (1984). 'Communicating with children', in *Paediatric Developmental Therapy*, pp. 53–62. LEVITT, S. (ed). Oxford: Blackwell.

LEVITT, S. (1984). 'The cerebral palsies', in *Paediatric Developmental Therapy*, pp. 110–126. LEVITT, S. (ed). Oxford: Blackwell.

MUELLER, H. (1974). 'Speech', in *Handling the Young Cerebral Palsied Child at Home*, pp. 131–138. FINNIE, N. R. (ed). London: Heinemann.

NASH, M. I. (1977). 'Assessment of gross and fine motor function in cerebral palsy', in *Neurodevelopmental Problems in Early Childhood*, pp. 166–174. DRILLIEN, C. and DRUMMOND, M. (eds). Oxford: Blackwell.

NOLAN, M. and TUCKER, I. G. (1988, 2nd Edition). *The Hearing Impaired Child and the Family*. London: Souvenir Press.

RUSSELL, P. (1984). *The Wheelchair Child*. London: Souvenir Press.

SCRUTTON, D. (1984). 'Aim-orientated management', in *Management of the Motor Disorders of Children with Cerebral Palsy*, pp.

49–58. SCRUTTON, D. (ed). Spastics International Medical Publications. Oxford: Blackwell; Philadelphia: Lippincott.

SYKANDA, A. M. and LEVITT, S. (1982). 'The physiotherapist in the developmental management of the visually impaired child', *Child: care, health and development*, **8**, 261–270.

WHITE, R. (1984). 'Sensory integration therapy for the cerebral palsied child', in *The Management of Motor Disorders in Cerebral Palsy*, pp. 86–95. SCRUTTON, D. (ed). Spastics International Medical Publications. Oxford: Blackwell; Philadelphia: Lippincott.

7   Education

Education shall be directed to the full development of the human personality

Universal Declaration of Human Rights
Article 26.1

This quotation was chosen for this chapter because it describes what the aim should be in the education of all children, and the objective throughout this book has been to promote the best for the 'whole' child.

It is generally agreed that in the choice of a school parents and administrators will have regard to finding a school that will be right for a particular child. Recent legislation in the United Kingdom is putting more and more stress on parent participation on governing bodies of schools, as well as on parental choice of schools for their own child. The grounds for such choice may be very variable; the school down the road because it is handy; a school further away because its examination results are good; the recommendation of a friend or acquaintance; family connections; religious grounds, and many others. Some choices do not always take full account of the child's individual aptitudes.

In the case of a child who has cerebral palsy the choice is often more difficult and may be limited as the question of his 'special needs' must be taken into account. Nearly all parents wish for their child with special educational needs to attend an ordinary school, but in addition to the criteria which parents use for their choice of an ordinary school must be added the question of whether the special needs will be fulfilled.

Hopefully the child's development during the pre-school years, the results of assessment revealing strengths and weaknesses, and the child's response to the help and support that has been given, will provide a sufficiently accurate picture of the child and his needs to enable his carers to find the best educational solution. This also requires a knowledge of the various types of school from which a suitable choice can be made.

In 1978 the Department of Education and Science issued the Warnock Report. Amongst its recommendations were multidisciplinary assessment; special importance of early intervention, including education; the introduction of the term 'special educational need'; the ending of categorisation for educational purposes; the importance of normal social contact; the integration of pupils with special educational needs into ordinary schools as much as possible.

The Education Act 1981

This Act, which was largely based upon the findings of the Warnock Report (1978) and the responses to the discussion paper 1980, promotes a statutory basis for the education of children who have special educational needs and requires that the local authority should, wherever possible, arrange for the child's education in an ordinary school where this is compatible with:

(a)   his receiving the special educational provision that he requires;

(b)   the provision of efficient education for the children with whom he will be educated;

(c)   the efficient use of resources.*

As the Act is concerned with all children who have special educational needs, those who have cerebral palsy are only a small proportion. Most children will therefore be educated in ordinary schools, but the Act also makes allowance for special schools either maintained by the local authority or approved independent schools (Ch. 60 para 11).

Integration
The child's needs
In an early paper considering handicapped children in ordinary schools Kershaw (1974) pointed out that a child's

* Chapter 60, paragraph 2(3).

special needs may be educational, social, emotional or therapeutic, and the present definition of special educational needs under the Act may be taken to encompass all four aspects in line with the Universal Declaration of Human Rights. It is therefore particularly important, when considering an individual child's special needs, to recognise the total difficulty that the child may experience in adjusting to a full life in an ordinary school. Kershaw suggests that the total powers of adaptation are often limited by physical difficulties and, further, that too much stress may increase the disability. In other words it is not sufficient to consider what theoretical benefits might accrue to a child by being in a normal school; it is essential to estimate the amount of extra physical effort that will be demanded of a child with cerebral palsy. In addition to needing a longer time to undertake some tasks, exhaustion may make the child less efficient than he need be, and failure will exacerbate feelings of inadequacy. Sensitivity to such problems will be needed on the part of all teachers.

It is clear that the best interest of each child requires a choice of school that can offer the type of education most suited to his/her needs, which should have been identified during assessment. For all children integration into mainstream schooling will be the aim, but for some children this may not be possible or desirable. The degree of physical handicap and the severity of learning difficulty are both obvious factors to take into consideration (Cope and Anderson, 1977), but in addition satisfactory adjustment to the school situation depends upon other characteristics of personality and circumstances. Bowley and Gardner (1980) sum these up as follows: 1) Good drive, persistence and resilience on the part of the child; 2) Parental support; 3) Special advice and attention to communication difficulties both early in life and throughout school; 4) A reasonable balance between overprotection and underprotection. These factors are reiterated again and again by other writers. It is generally accepted that a child's outgoing personality and resilience (O'Moore, 1980; Hegarty et al,

1981; Madge and Fassam, 1982) are most important in generating popularity and acceptance by other children. This is also related to independence which needs to be fostered both at home and at school. Hegarty and his colleagues (1981) enumerate such details as having high expectations, giving pupils responsibility, allowing them to take risks, making a minimum of interventions and concessions, and above all firm discipline, thus steering a middle course between over- and underprotection, and giving a reminder to parents and professionals of the value of these attributes in early intervention. These principles need to be followed in both ordinary and special schools, and will certainly require close co-operation, understanding and consistency between parents, teachers and other professionals. Madge and Fassam (1982) found that children themselves who were asked emphasised all these points (to which the authors would add the importance of adequate assessment and provision of resources).

The schools
The importance of the right choice of school for each individual child requires knowledge of the schools just as much as knowledge of the children. The processes by which the children's needs can be evaluated have been considered in some detail, but after this careful procedure the choice of school is occasionally somewhat arbitrary.

If consideration is to be given to the full development of the child's personality, with respect to his special needs, certain criteria need to be considered (Cope and Anderson 1977; Kershaw, 1974): a) educational aspects, b) physical and medical needs, c) the social environment, and d) the extent of integration. The educational aspects should fall within the boundaries of the school curriculum, unless the child has special learning difficulties. Medical and physical needs may require extra resources and will be discussed later. The social environment is probably the most important in helping children to maturity, and integration may be effected in a number of different ways, as follows:

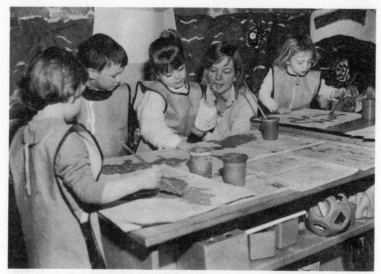

Plate 8   Integration. This little girl with 'special needs' is enjoying a painting session with her peers.

1.   Full integration into an ordinary school without any additional help or special allowances. This is the ideal which can be accomplished by some individuals whose future will follow the same lines as other children in the school, and who will mature with them, form friendships as equals and find success in their own fields.

2.   Children who have moderate or severe difficulty in mobility and manipulation but no other problems may need a little extra help from ancillary staff (Plate 8), but otherwise can be absorbed into all normal school activities and the additional help may be gradually withdrawn. If children are actively mobile in wheelchairs, simple structural alterations may need to be made to accommodate them (p. 114).

3.   At the secondary school level a special unit for physically handicapped pupils may provide for a group of children of mixed ages and handicaps who can take part in

whole school activities selected for their individual aptitudes and interests.

4.   A special school for physically handicapped children
may be sited adjacent to an ordinary primary, middle or
secondary school and shared activities may be arranged, in
which pupils from each school may attend certain lessons
together.

5.   For cerebral palsied children who have learning,
other sensory difficulties or epilepsy, or who are very
limited in their movements, learning requirements may be
so complicated that a fully specialised curriculum and
environment may be needed in a special school for the
physically handicapped.

6.   If children are severely mentally handicapped a
special care unit within a special school (for either physically or mentally handicapped pupils) will be the most
probable solution.

Integration needs to be realistic, and where it can be
achieved within the first three categories above is far and
away the most satisfactory for cerebral palsied children and
their normal peers. However, these are not necessarily easy
options and are certainly no more economic than special
schools, but the reward on the whole is greater. It is
essential for success that the child who has cerebral palsy
should be welcomed by the head, the teachers and the
other children, and that these teachers who will be involved
with the child should have been fully briefed about his
difficulties in any field, and should be encouraged to treat
him like other children. It is normally expected that the
school doctor and school nurse will provide full explanations without breaching any special requirements for
confidentiality.

The necessity for admission to a special school should
never be considered 'second best', and annual review
should ensure that transfer to mainstream education can be
effected later if the child's progress warrants it, and if
specialised teaching techniques and/or fairly intensive
medical or therapeutic care are no longer essential.

Check List

Many teachers or head teachers who have not previously admitted cerebral palsied children into their classes or school, may be at a loss, at first, to know what to expect of the child or what questions to ask the mother. Table 2 gives a suggested simple check list so that the teacher can know what the child can or cannot perform and can ask for advice from the school doctor or nurse or community therapist as to how a particular problem can be dealt with.

Resources Needed to Meet the Physical Needs of Cerebral Palsied Children Attending Ordinary Schools

Planning the admission of a child with a physical handicap to an ordinary school should be started long before the child enters the school. This planning should include the necessary alteration of buildings, the choosing of equipment and furniture, and advisory discussions with the teacher and head teacher as to the problems which that child might present as he is integrated into the school.

Buildings and access   For any child to gain the maximum from his surroundings, he must be able to relate to them, feel at ease, negotiate them and above all feel safe in them. With these things catered for he will have a secure backdrop for his educational and social learning. At the same time the planners must remember that any alterations needed should be kept to the minimum as it is important for the child to integrate and learn to cope in a normal living situation.

Areas of consideration are ramps beside, or in place of, steps, handrails along walls, particularly toilet and washing areas, and non-slip flooring, again particularly in areas which might be wet or damp. A wider toilet cubicle, to allow for a wheelchair, will lead to independence. Showers in the games area may need a seat and a sloping floor instead of a stand-in cubicle. In some cases some sort of chair lift would be needed to allow for independent negotiation of a flight of stairs, and one area may need to be set aside for the recharging of electric wheelchairs. Door

Table 2. Suggested Check List for the Admission of Handicapped Children into Mainstream Schools

1. *Mobility* Using any means (including wheelchair), can child, given time, move from desk (or equivalent) to toilet, to dining/assembly hall, to other classrooms, to playground? Can he/she take part in PE, art, drama, music, etc? (If not, is environment the cause and can it be altered?) Is he/she safe in playground? Can he/she manage stairs? How will he/she come to school?

2. *Vision* Has it been tested? Does child need to wear glasses? for distance? for close work? Does child need special equipment, e.g. magnifying glass, large print, telescopic lens? Should child be seated in special place in class?

3. *Hearing* Has it been tested recently? Does it fluctuate? Does child wear a hearing aid? (If so, staff need to know how it works.) Is a radio loop system necessary?

4. *Manipulation* Can child handle pencil, crayon, etc? Buttons and fastenings? Cutlery? Books? Other equipment?

5. *Intelligence* This entails multidisciplinary assessment and often a period of observation of the child's response to help offered. Formal IQ testing may be of little value in children with senosry or performance problems.

6. *Communication* (This will be affected by any defect in hearing.) Is expressive speech adequate and intelligible? Is comprehension within normal limits? Does he/she use other methods of communication?

7. *Social Skills* Feeding, dressing, washing, toilet, etc. Is help needed?

8. *Behaviour* (Children with handicaps may have these problems, just as ordinary children, but it is important to sort out whether the handicap is contributing significantly and whether additional help is needed.) Is the child excessively quiet? Lonely? Withdrawn? Sulky? Non-co-operative? Sad? Happy? Willing?

9. *Specific Learning Difficulties* These are probably no more common in children with handicaps than in others but are more difficult to identify, and will need special help when discovered.

10. *Relationships* With family? With adults? With other children?

11. *Epilepsy* Is the child known to have convulsions? If so, is he on medication? Does it need to be given at school?

12. Is he on any other medication?

widths and handle heights usually accommodate wheelchairs, but the children will need to learn how to negotiate
the heavier fire safety doors (Eckersley et al, 1986).

Under the title of access, transport arrangements to and
from the school must be included. The Education Authority
should provide suitable transport arrangements. This
usually means a school bus with adaptations to convey
wheelchairs and pupils in line with safety regulations as
laid down by the Ministry of Transport. The bus will
normally also be fitted with a tail lift.

Furniture and equipment   As much use as possible should be
made of standard school furniture. However, heights of
work-benches in such areas as science laboratories and
home economics kitchens may need some changes to allow
for the physically handicapped child's needs. With both
sitting and standing activities it is important that the child
should work at the same height as his peers whenever
possible. For this reason it is important he does not remain
all the time in his wheelchair, but moves to an ordinary
classroom chair and table. If his balance is poor then arms
may be required on the chair. In a busy classroom it is very
easy to knock and be knocked by someone.

Standing at a work bench he may be helped by handrails
or a simple standing frame. Non-slip table mats may be
used in many activities, e.g. to hold paper on desk tops
aiding writing, and to hold a plate at lunch time.

Equipment needed by the visiting community therapist
for treatment purposes can usually be found in the gym-
nasium, e.g. mats. More specific things like hoists and
hydraulic beds to aid toileting may also be useful.

Personal equipment   The child's personal equipment may
include walking aids, shoes, splints, a cycle, cushions, etc.
Advice about these and their uses should be given to the
teachers and helpers by the therapist.

Any children who have additional disabilities may need
to bring other personal equipment to school. Children with
visual problems may need to use large magnifying glasses,

or video screens for reading, and may need to be seated at the front of the class. Blackboards are particularly difficult for some children with poor sight. Teachers need to make sure that children who have been issued with glasses wear them regularly. Children with hearing impairment also need to be at the front of the class to enable them to use their skill at lip-reading, and it is very advisable that the teacher should understand how a hearing aid works and how to make sure that it is functioning properly. A microphone for the teacher with a small radio transmitter and a receiving unit for the child may greatly improve the child's ability to function in the classroom and may be passed from teacher to teacher with the child carrying his receiving set (Nolan and Tucker, 1988).

Children who have difficulty with speech may need to use other methods of communication. Sign language is not always possible for them and they may need to use pointing with the index finger (or a stick) at symbols (before they can read), as in Blissymbolics system (Latham, 1984), and later using a board on which letters, numbers and common words are printed. If severe difficulties in writing are encountered due to poor manual dexterity, a typewriter should be used as soon as the child is able to read and wishes to express ideas in writing.

Advisory Role of the External Professions
Integration of children with cerebral palsy can be greatly helped by advice and in-service training from the visiting health care team. The paediatric physiotherapist will be one of the people who will have the knowledge to advise the teachers on the child's physical capabilities and will provide liaison between the school and parents to promote greater independence in the pupils (Hegarty et al, 1981).

The growing importance of the child's education will necessitate the gradual withdrawal of the therapeutic input. However, the importance of therapy must not go unrecognised but should become a more integrated part of the child's day. This may prove viable by the training of ancillary staff, such as the nursery nurse in an 'enhanced' classroom. She can be trained in the simple basic tasks of handling the child to promote greater independence and should always be seen as a member of the classroom staff available to help the whole group in a number of ways.

Physical education is important, and the PE teacher and physiotherapist can collaborate in devising activities in which the whole class can participate (George and Hart, 1983). Swimming is another beneficial activity and mildly disabled children can take part in ordinary swimming sessions; those with a more severe handicap may need to learn in a warmer pool. Horse-riding is usually on the curriculum of special schools, but more difficult to arrange for children in mainstream schools.

'Statements'

Any child who has Special Educational Needs will have a statement drawn up as a result of the assessment findings. Contributions to the Statement include parental evidence, educational advice, medical advice and psychological advice. Where there has been fruitful interdisciplinary co-operation these sets of advice will include the findings of individual members of the assessment team, and will thus provide a true and multidimensional picture of the child's abilities and difficulties, which will form the basis of the education authority's recommendation. The parents may need help in preparing their evidence and may look to their key worker for this. The professional advice needs to be in simple non-technical terms and should express the difficulties a child will experience on entering a school, and describe the extra resources that will be needed. At least two years before the end of his school life, it is necessary to begin a realistic appraisal of a child's competence in the many fields of endeavour he will need in adult life. Review and provision of a leaving statement will be required but, more than this, careers staff will need to search for placement that will offer full development of the individual's personality.

As long ago as 1970, Younghushand and her colleagues expressed concern for the future of disabled school leavers as follows: 'The school curriculum, especially in the last year, should give due consideration to the need for preparation for life after school, particularly personal independence, social relationships and pre-work experience.' It is essential that these aims should be kept in view, not only from the child's first entry into school, but from the time that the disability was first recognised.

Conductive Education
In view of the present (1988) interest in the value of Conductive Education some readers may wonder why it has not been enthusiastically advocated as 'the only' or even 'the best' system of helping children who have cerebral palsy. Other readers may have observed references in the text to some of its principles such as the importance of group dynamics, considering the child as a whole, encouragement of every small success and motivation towards independence. Many of these principles and useful items of furniture have been incorporated into the British less totalitarian approach for many years (Levitt, 1984).

We would like to make it clear that although we agree with some of its dicta, which are similar to ours, we do not believe that exclusive use of methods which apparently have been successful in Hungary would be as appropriate to the population of cerebral palsied children in Great Britain and other countries in the West. Our reasons are as follows:

a) We need to provide a comprehensive service to benefit all children who have cerebral palsy, however severely they are affected. This entails making flexible use of all possible approaches to treatment and education that are suitable for the individual;

b) We believe that help for children should be provided as nearly as possible to their own home, and that wherever possible children should attend their local school (1981 Education Act), whether they are able to walk or not. We usually find it almost impossible to form the 'homogenous' groups that are so essential and indeed easy to produce in such an institutionalised residential approach as Conductive Education.

c) In view of the interesting and worthwhile post-school lives evidenced in those young people we contacted (see Chapter 8), we consider that the present services available for people with cerebral palsy as described in these chapters, if expanded, will be successful in fulfilling the lives of cerebral palsied people as whole persons. In particular we consider the needs of those young persons who will never be able fully to use their limbs or their voice. Some, whose brains are lively, are now able to live lives that are independent and fulfilled with the aid of technical and personal help; others who are more handicapped are being provided with ancillary help so that they need never be institutionalised.

References

BOWLEY, A. H. and GARDNER, L. (1980). *The Handicapped Child. Educational and Psychological Guidance for the Organically Handicapped*. Edinburgh: Churchill Livingstone.

COPE, C. and ANDERSON, E. (1977). *Special Units in Ordinary Schools*. London: University of London Institute of Education.

DEPARTMENT OF EDUCATION AND SCIENCE (1978). *Special Educational Needs. Report of the committee of enquiry into the education of children and young people. (The Warnock report)* London: HMSO

ECKERSLEY, P., CLEGG, M. and ROBINSON, P. (1986). *The 1981 Education Act. Guidelines for Physiotherapists and other Paediatric Professionals*. London: Chartered Society of Physiotherapy.

GEORGE, S. J. and HART, B. (1983). *Physical Education for Handicapped Children*. London: Souvenir Press.

HEGARTY, S. and POCKLINGTON, K. with LUCAS, D. (1981). *Educating Pupils with Special Needs in Ordinary Schools*. Windsor: NFER—Nelson.

KERSHAW, J. D. (1974). 'Handicapped Children in Ordinary

Schools' in *The Handicapped Person in the Community*, pp. 203–216. BOSWELL, D. M. and WINGROVE, J. M. (eds). London: Tavistock Publications and Open University.

LATHAM, C. (1984). 'Communicating with children' in *Paediatric Developmental Therapy*, pp. 53–62. LEVITT, S. (ed). Oxford: Blackwell.

LEVITT, S. (1984). *Paediatric Developmental Therapy*. Oxford: Blackwell.

MADGE, N. and FASSAM, M. (1982). *Ask the Children. Experiences of Disability in the School Years*. London: Batsford Academic and Educational Ltd.

NOLAN, M. and TUCKER, I. G. (1988, 2nd Edition). *The Hearing Impaired Child and the Family*. London: Souvenir Press.

O'MOORE, M. (1980). 'Social acceptance of the physically handicapped child in the ordinary school', *Child: care, health and development*, **6**, 317–337.

YOUNGHUSBAND, E., BIRCHALL, D., DAVIE, R. and PRINGLE, M. L. K. (1970). *Living with handicap*. London: National Bureau for Co-operation in Child Care.

8   After School

The Child is father of the Man

W. Wordsworth

Growing up brings its problems to able and disabled alike. Such terms as 'standing on one's own feet', 'making one's way in the world' emphasise the additional challenge that young people who have cerebral palsy will face.

It is accepted that some developmental needs and social problems are common to all adolescents although Morgan (1974) points out that these are not always recognised as being important or relevant as far as handicapped young people are concerned. She mentions in particular five aspects to be taken into consideration: 1. Identity and self determination; 2. Independence; 3. Respect (the need to be valued for onself); 4. Work and appropriate outlets for self expression; 5. Satisfactory relations with the opposite sex. Although these are factors which come into prominence at adolescence and particularly on leaving school they are not always catered for adequately in the school curriculum (as emphasised by Younghusband et al, 1970). It is worth taking note of these requirements even earlier than school life, i.e. during the early intervention phase, particularly in building up the child's self-image and self confidence. Morgan's five points are strongly supported by further research (e.g. Anderson et al, 1982; Hegarty et al, 1981; Brimblecombe, 1987), and need to be considered in greater depth.

1.   Identity and self-determination. Such questions as 'Who am I?', 'Where am I going?', 'What of the future?', are very real to adolescents (and are answered in a variety of ways). The young person who has cerebral palsy not only finds it difficult to express these questions, let alone find answers, but has additional ones such as 'Why am I like this?' and may feel guilty that it may be punishment for his own faults. These young people need explanation and

reassurance, that they are not odd, or different, or to blame for their situation. Very often professionals and even parents who are so committed to helping the person's difficulties which make him disabled, forget that in emotional terms he is the same as everyone else. Parents themselves are not always the people best able to give the information and encouragement needed, partly because they are so emotionally involved and also because they may not understand the implications of their child's condition. It may not be necessary to go to the length of suggesting genetic counselling but an understanding and sympathetic professional should be able to offer the counselling that is needed. Cope and Anderson (1977) see a role for the school nurse in this.

2. Independence. Morgan points out that even for ordinary young people strong drive and sometimes intense battles are needed to obtain independence, so how much more difficult this must be for handicapped young people. Independence needs to be encouraged from early childhood and it is difficult sometimes for parents and professionals, who are anxious to help the young child to make the most of his potential, to remember not only to allow but also to encourage every possible step to independence. Tantrums and refusals which are norms of development in all children, are much easier to repress in children who have cerebral palsy, whereas they may indicate early steps towards independence and their cause should be heeded. From replies of school children themselves (Cope and Anderson, 1977; Hegarty et al, 1981; Madge and Fassam, 1982) it appears that integration into mainstream schooling helps independence so long as children are encouraged to fend for themselves and are subject to the same disciplines.

3. The need to feel valued for themselves. This problem is exacerbated in disabled young people, partly because every activity is more difficult for them and partly through lack of popularity. This is one aspect of which class teachers and even parents are often unaware (O'Moore, 1980) and all need to be more sensitive to finding and praising the

things which children *can* do and fostering their self-confidence and friendliness in their relations with other children. All this is a preparation for later independence and should not be left for innovation on leaving school. Both girls and boys need to be encouraged to take an interest in their appearance and their apparel.

4. Work and appropriate outlets for self expression. This addresses the question of careers advice, and the correct step and placement immediately on leaving school. Most children who have cerebral palsy will have a 'Statement' whether they are attending an ordinary or special school, and for these children review at the age of 12½–13½ is mandatory; for others it is certainly advisable. And from then on realistic appraisal of a child's academic attainments, physical disability, social competence and personality is needed, so that the right one of the many alternatives can be selected for each individual after the age of 16 years.

The full range of possibilities is very adequately explored in a publication from the Family Fund (Glendinning et al, 1987), which furnishes full details of all possible avenues for education, work and training and for financial assistance. However, it is worthwhile here to consider an outline of the paths available to young people, and to take time and thought and consultation for each individual.

Education   Although many young people leave school at the age of 16 years all have the right to stay until their 19th birthday. In mainstream education most of the pupils who stay on into sixth forms or enter sixth form colleges do so with the purpose of taking further examinations and going on to higher education. This may be the case for some children who have cerebral palsy who may go straight on to University or Polytechnic. Less intellectually gifted children, whose need for continuing education is just as great, may find it difficult to fit into this pattern. For them, as for many of those who leave school at 16, admission to a College of Further Education may be the solution, where they can follow either general courses improving basic educational skills, academic courses preparing for GCSE and other examinations, or vocational courses leading to skilled employment. However, not all cerebral palsied young people will be ready for this and they may require bridging courses which are designed to ease the transition from school to further education and employment or special courses which are specifically geared to foster skills for independent living. Participation in courses provided for able bodied students may thus become possible later.

Employment   Few young people who have cerebral palsy are ready to enter paid employment in the open market at the age of 16, but they can, like their able bodied peers, take part in Youth Training Schemes. Entry to these is open to young people aged 16 (for two years) or 17 (normally for one year) but handicapped applicants are accepted for two years up to the age of 21, and may be allowed an extra six months for training or assessment if it is deemed necessary. Following these training schemes young people may go on to open or sheltered employment.

Other options   Some young adults who have cerebral palsy are too handicapped, physically, mentally, or multiply to be able to take part in further education or any type of employment. Some, with a minimal or moderate physical disability but with marked impairment of learning, may attend Adult Training Centres which are run for people with severe learning difficulties. When the physical disability is more severe, special units within adult training centres or special day centres may be chosen.

Leisure activities   These are important for everyone, and possibly even more important for those whose choice of life-style or scope to chose their daily employment is limited. Sport of all kinds not only makes life more exhilarating but also has beneficial effects on physical development and self confidence. Young people who enjoyed swimming, horse riding or athletics at school should be encouraged and helped to find outlets for their chosen activity, and perhaps enabled to explore such sports as canoeing, sailing, skiing and mountain climbing, any of which may be catered for by one or other of the voluntary societies. Music, drama and art can all be enjoyed through television and radio, but like sporting leisure activities are much more worthwhile if people are enabled to participate. Table tennis, snooker, darts or chess are excellent activities for the less athletic.

Health requirements   One of the hazards of leaving school where special support services were always available is the sudden cessation of these provisions. Paediatric surveillance, the advice and encouragement of therapists, social workers and teachers are no longer part of the every day scene, and the young person and his parents are all on their own. Although developmental therapy is no longer needed it is still possible for deformities to occur, so that some continuing contact with therapeutic facilities is desirable. Vision testing, dentistry, and so on have to be sought and financial hurdles dealt with. Aids and appliances still need supervision and changing as new inventions come forward and the young person continues to grow.

Assessment   The need is still present although the teams will be different. It has been emphasised time and again that assessment is a continuous process, particularly as the needs for support and advice change. Assessment must always be realistic with regard to the person's skills at the time and the development of other skills in the future, bearing in mind not only any physical and other disabilities but also drive and motivation, ability to make relationships and the support of the environment. Although parents still continue to have a keen interest and continuing responsibility, the young person on reaching the age of 16 should be encouraged to speak for himself and to define his own needs within the limits of his disability. This will then lead on to a mutual decision as to the next step, and during this first post-school placement the responses to various challenges, educational and social situations, and the burgeoning of maturity and independence, will be a guide to the next step and so on, until a progressive and productive niche has been found.

5. Satisfactory relations with the opposite sex. Morgan wrote at a time when very little consideration was being given to the emotional needs of young handicapped people, hence her emphasis is on opposite sexes. However, later research (e.g. Anderson et al, 1980; Hegarty et al, 1981) has revealed that cerebral palsied young people may have difficulty in forming friendships and making relationships with either sex. So far the reasons for this are undefined, although quite clearly uncertainty as to personal identity, lack of self-confidence and the bugbear of young adolescents' self-consciousness about their personal appearance, may all be factors. It is uncertain whether the root cause lies in knowledge of the disabilities, in the need for being cared for, the lack of opportunities to make choices and to determine their own actions or a combination of these and other problems, but it is quite clear that there are limiting factors in forming human relationships for many handicapped young people. It may be that increasing opportunities for independence and the fostering from an early age of a good and positive self image may change this situation.

Fortunately the increasing mixing of boys and girls in mainstream and special education is enabling young people of both sexes to meet and share experiences. Even now parents and professionals are nervous of any 'serious' relationships developing, although for most of us the emotional aspect of our lives is the most precious and, hopefully, the most enduring. Part of this reluctance may be related to fears that offspring might be affected, too, but cerebral palsy is not an inherited condition, and society should try to support disabled young people to enjoy, if they so wish, relationships that are the very basis of our humanity, to share one another's lives and to have children if they are able to bring them up. Sex and sexuality is still, so often, a taboo subject and not always easy to discuss with parents. Shearer (1974) makes some very helpful comments on this subject. Disabled youngsters need a good deal of reassurance that love and affection are available to all, although its expression may vary considerably, and beauty is always in the eye of the beholder.

From the outset the essential diversity and complexity of the effects of cerebral palsy has been emphasised and nowhere is it more clearly seen than in the consideration of adolescents and young adults. All the earlier detailed considerations of early intervention, assessment, 'treatment' and education have been leading up to the chance for the person to find his identity, develop independence, and take pleasure in personal relationships. We still have a long way to go and it will *never* be easy.

To illustrate the diversity of persons and prospects, we have invited some young people, we think a random but representative sample, whom we knew as young children to tell us and our readers of their experiences and hopes for the future. By chance, between them, they cover almost all the points raised in this chapter; and those who have attained independence certainly outline the pleasure and fulfilment that it brings. We thank them for their help.

Jean writes as follows:

> Between the ages of 11 and 17 I attended Penn Secondary Modern School with normal school curriculum. I remember very little about my school days.
>
> When not at school I lived with my parents and twin brother, John (10 minutes the younger). My upbringing was strict but we had a happy childhood. At home I was treated as a normal child—not a disabled child.
>
> On leaving school I started work at Contactor Switchgear-Electronics Ltd. My job there was Printed Circuit Board Inspection. During my 17 years at the firm the company was taken over three times, and name changed twice. I was the sole survivor of the Electronics Division. Also my job changed to Catalogue Clerk, which continued up until I left to have my eldest child, Helen, in December 1981.
>
> In between times I started going to the Smiling Faces

Youth Club, when it started up in 1965. I took an active part in the running of the club. At one time I took the part of Secretary of the youth club.

I met my husband, Brian, shortly after the start up of the club. Brian is not disabled. We started going out together in 1968. Brian was working away from home at the time—in Anglesey—we got engaged in 1969 on my birthday in October. Our wedding day, May 1971, was nice weather and well attended, and we still believe everyone—including ourselves—had a happy and enjoyable day.

The children came along in 1982 and 1984, both natural births. Owing to lack of feeling in my left side, the only labour pains occurred during the actual delivery—about 20 minutes—in both births. Helen is our eldest and up until I had her I had never even held a baby, but here I was looking after one all day long. She was a good baby and still loves being cuddled. She can also sleep amongst a lot of noise, so if she is asleep we do not bother tip-toeing around or whispering.

Neil was not too bad as a baby, except when he was born the midwife found a tiny hole in the middle of his back. At six months old he underwent an operation to seal up this hole at Birmingham Children's Hospital. Up until then we could not give him a proper bath, just wash him down. How he loves a bath.

Neil is registered hyperactive. He has blonde hair, blue eyes and long eyelashes coupled with a cheeky smile. The looks of an angel but the mischievousness of an imp.

As Neil is hyperactive and a handful I have to have a girl helping me five mornings a week to help with the housework.

Both of us work together in all things to do with the bringing up of our children, and they are showing signs of being very independent.

In April 1986 I became a member of the Midlands

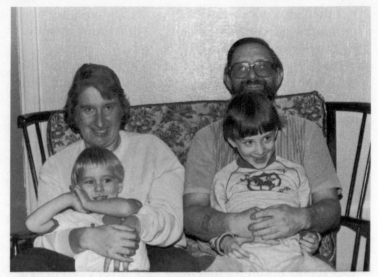

Plate 9   Jean with her husband Brian and their two children, Helen (5) and Neil (3).

Region Alpha Advisory Committee to the Spastics
Society.

Jan types for herself:

'I will have to go in a minute, I am in the middle of
cooking my tea,' I said to my friend who had just
phoned me. This is a typical statement to make when
one is cooking a meal, and the phone rings. It is,
however, unusual to be using another pair of arms and
legs to cook the meal, and using the voice which
belongs to the pair of arms and legs to speak on the
telephone. This is an example of the independence I
can now enjoy, even though I am a person with severe
disabilities, needing total physical help. In this article
I hope to explain how this independence can be
achieved.

I am a woman in my mid-thirties and I have cerebral palsy. I use an electric wheelchair to get about, and my method of communication is by a word board. Until eighteen months ago I lived with my parents who had always treated me as normal, giving me every opportunity to live as full and active a life as my disabilities would allow. It is for this reason I had dreaded the time when I would have to enter a Home for people with disabilities when my parents could no longer look after me.

Three years ago my parents and I decided it was time for me to leave home. My social worker came to see me to talk over the question of residential homes, and which one would suit me. She told me about a newly opened hostel for people with disabilities in Kidderminster, three miles from my home village, and recommended I should go to see the officer in charge. This is what I duly did to talk over the possibility of the hostel being suitable for me. The philosophy behind the running of the hostel is unusual in that we, the residents, are in control of our own lives mentally, and the staff are our arms and legs to carry out the physical tasks to independence.

Let me now describe the hostel. It has four levels —level 1 is the basement, levels 2 and 3 are living accommodation for people with disabilities and level 4 has offices, a laundry room, and a big community space. I live on level 2 with three other permanent residents, and quite often a short-stay resident. I have a good-sized bedsitter, with my own toilet attached, and my own outside door leading onto a verandah. I share a kitchen with my fellow residents living on level 2, and there is a communal bath and shower room we all use.

With the staff here as my arms and legs for physically doing the things I cannot do for myself, I am responsible for every aspect of my lifestyle and welfare. I decide for myself what time I would like to get up in the morning, what time I would like my meals, and what food to eat. I am responsible for buying my own food and budgeting my money accordingly.

We lead very different lifestyles on the level. I like to keep myself occupied in my bedsitter most of the day, appearing in our communal area for drinks and meals. I spend many hours at my electric typewriter writing letters, doing various typing jobs for people, writing poetry and keeping a diary. Apart from typing I enjoy reading and being creative with my one hand, knitting, tapestry work or weaving on a loom.

I am lucky enough to have my own car here at the hostel. It is an adapted Escort van which takes me sitting in my chair. Although I cannot drive, the car is insured so that other people can drive for me. I am a Christian and belong to a church in Kidderminster. I can book staff time to drive me to church on a Sunday evening and to pick me up again after the service. Likewise on a Wednesday evening I go to a fellowship meeting and can arrange staff help to get there and back. Apart from these weekly trips out, I go to a day centre in Birmingham once a week, and have a good social life outside the hostel.

In this article I hope I have given some idea of how independently, I can live, using other people's arms and legs. I find it both challenging and satisfying to be in control of my own life. What is challenging is remembering to do the little things which make life run smoothly—when I see my medication getting low I have to remember to get a repeat prescription from my doctor, or remembering on a Thursday night to put my money ready for the milkman. What is satisfying is being able to decide for myself how I want to live—if I am having a busy day, and only want an apple for lunch for quickness nobody says I should eat a proper meal. It is also satisfying to be able to entertain friends in my bedsitter to coffee or even a meal that I have planned and directed how it should be cooked.

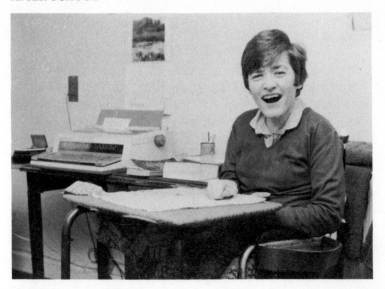

Plate 10   Jan, 1987.

It is my sincere hope that in the future more people with severe disabilities will be able to live as independent a life as I enjoy now, and the more traditional residential homes will adopt the philosophy behind the running of this hostel. As I have mentioned, I am a Christian and I believe Jesus would approve of this philosophy of giving the people with disabilities the right to have complete control over their lives, instead of people to be looked after in a way other people think best.

This extract is taken from an article in *The Residential And Day Care Weekly*, October 30th, 1987 by the permission of the author (Jan) and publishers.

Ruth (29) writes as follows:

My first experience of school was in the nursery department of a special school for children with cerebral palsy, and my memory only extends to the taxi journeys to and from school.

At an ordinary Primary and Junior School I did reasonably well, although failed to get entrance to the grammar school. I took part in all the lessons, although experienced difficulties with swimming and music lessons. Here, because of co-ordination problems, I could only master certain percussion instruments, although I was bought a recorder to see if I could manage. Regrettably, the form teacher did not appreciate the situation. At needlework I was slow, and the whole process was rather fiddly. It was during my time at Woodfield I was told I was a spastic and incurable. I soon learned not to be open about it and to expect difficulties, if not taunts. This has a positive side—had I attended a 'special' school I wouldn't have been so teased, nor had 'my edges hardened' so early, thus making me more able to cope.

At my Dominican Convent School I participated fully in school life, although once again finding needlework difficult. In other practical areas, sports and cookery, I had little exemptions—not enough to be called specialist attention and for the most part had exactly the same conditions as my peers. My cookery teacher apparently had not been aware she had a spastic in the form—communication between her and the headmistress had faltered.

I enjoyed most of my sports and on one occasion played hockey for the school—and on another for the House so was by-and-large judged on the same standard. We were given lessons in public speaking which has helped me verbally to explain my spasticity and its effects, invaluable in all situations as confidence breeds confidence.

I left with three 'O' level passes.

At the Wulfrun College of Further Education I enrolled for a two-year course in basic office skills. The end examination was a Certificate of Office Studies only attained if five or so of the amalgam of subjects taken were passed. The Course offered a total of about eight subjects.

The syllabus included familiar subjects, e.g. Economic History, English and Mathematics, together with the office-related typing, shorthand and commerce lessons. There was the chance to take 'O' level and other examinations together with the Certificate.

I started in September and by January it was clear my spasticity wasn't allowing me to improve in typing past 37 wpm, insufficient for any examinations. The course tutors were considerate enough to join together in a personalised syllabus the commerce, accounting and other academic subjects of both first and second year courses for me alone. I therefore dropped typing and shorthand to make room for the extra work. I was therefore a year early with my examinations but was successful not only in the Certificate but in other examinations I took simultaneously. It was from this springboard, and on such a positive upturn, that I joined the Department of Health and Social Security.

Largely this was not a happy experience, a classic case of what cannot be seen (my spasticity) cannot exist.

It was promotion which allowed me to transfer to the Metropolitan Police in 1979 where I still work on the Civil Staff, competing under exactly the same procedures for promotion boards and annual reports.

Spastics' Games

My involvement in the Spastics' Games began in 1969 and lasted until 1974. The Games allowed me to compete on equal terms, to find events I could master, to spend whole days without having to explain away one's limp or curled hand. I was successful and have several awards to remember the competitions by. I am still proud of having represented Great Britain twice, and in a total of ten track and field events. The initial exhilaration of winning is a remarkable experience and years afterwards, I can point to an actual achievement.

The Games gave me an aggression, a will to win, and appreciation of how little my difficulties are.

I will never cease to be periodically frustrated over being spastic. Problems vary, and what I can achieve today was a problem once. Frustration is not concerned with any particular difficulty although it may surface because of some. Frustration is against the disability and its permanence and 'coming to terms' is relative. Paradoxically I almost have to remind myself I

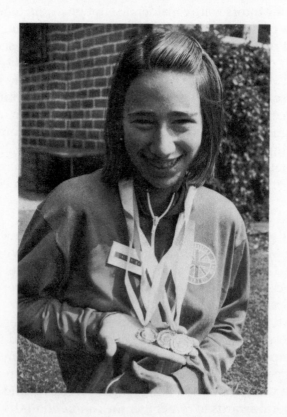

Plate 11   Ruth with her three gold medals won at European Spastics Games, 1972. (*Reproduced by permission of Wolverhampton Express and Star.*)

am spastic, such is the slight nature of my spasticity, mainly in order not to take on too much.

I have happily reached the stage where it doesn't matter to others or to my own confidence that I am spastic—I can hold my own.

Nigel (25) has a hearing impairment and learning difficulties as well as cerebral palsy. He attended a residential school and after that a unit for extended education in daily living. He was glad to come home to his mother (who still spoils him!) and his stepfather. He has brothers and sisters in the neighbourhood, attends the local ATC and is a great favourite in the local pub. He can walk a certain distance, although rather unsteadily, and he has no complaints!

Richard (23) and Joanna (22) live in the same community as Jan. Visiting them all three together was an occasion for fun and laughter. Joanna is the talkative one; she described her recent visit to Canada, and the way she formed a Dial-a-Taxi service for the residents and managed to fund it by organising, in the neighbourhood, a wheelchair sponsored walk. Richard has more difficulty with speech, and he is the Fire Officer.

All three are sure that what they appreciate most is their independence from home (although they all have caring and supportive families) and consider themselves very fortunate to live in a unit which has no counterpart in England outside London.

William types as follows:

I spent two years at Beaumont College in Lancaster, where I learnt to be much more independent and self-sufficient than I had been. I was surprised that some things which I learnt to do were much easier than I expected, e.g. shopping on my own and preparing the food that I had bought. We used microwave ovens for cooking which I found very quick and safe, and I was able to buy lots of different ready-made meals, which I put in the microwave for a few minutes, and I had a whole meal.

I enjoyed the walking weekends in the Lake District and sometimes we camped, which I had never done before. As a result of enjoying this activity, I am going to join our Local Rambling Club, which meets once a month and does a 10–12 mile walk in our lovely local countryside.

I left Beaumont in July 1987 and for the last two months I have been at Evesham College, where I am doing a two-year YTS skills course. I am learning a lot of different skills, some of which are decorating, welding, carpentry and cooking. At the moment, I am finding most of these things very difficult, as my eyesight is poor and I am unable to use my right hand, and so I am not enjoying it very much, but I realise it is early days and am hopeful that I will find it easier in time.

William Chesterson

Simon types as follows:

I left school when I was 17 and went to Beaumont College in Lancaster which is a College of Further Education for the Physically Handicapped.

I shared a room with my friend William who I was at school with and at first I was very unhappy. All I wanted to do was to come home again but Mum and Dad made me stay for 3 weeks before I came home, I then didn't want to go back again and for the first 2 terms I was very unhappy about going back after holidays.

After this everything was a lot better and I made a lot of friends from all over the Country. The staff were very kind and we had to learn to think for ourselves and ask

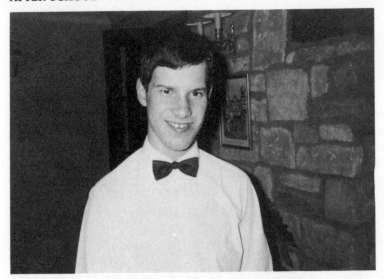

Plate 12   William.

for any help we needed. I enjoyed the Computer work
and the Independent Living Unit where we had to go
shopping for our food and cook it. We also had to do
our own washing and ironing. I enjoyed several outings to football matches, including a visit to Wembley,
cricket matches and wrestling.

The Second Year at College I really enjoyed. I had a
room to myself next door to my best friend Mike from
Liverpool. We both support Liverpool football club. I
was awarded the Duke of Edinburgh Bronze Award at
the end of the course and also several swimming
certificates. I was very happy there and would have
liked to go back for another year but it was only a 2 year
course.

In September this year (1987) I started a Bridging
Course at Evesham College of Education. This is a
course for further education and also mixing with able

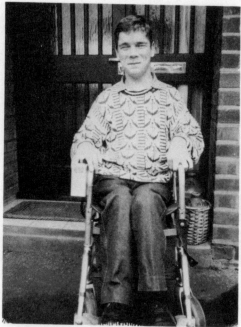

Plate 13   Simon.

bodied students. I am really enjoying it. We had a week at a holiday bungalow in Barmouth a fortnight ago. There were 7 students and 3 staff and we cooked for ourselves. We also had a visit down a slate mine. This is a course for 2 years and I don't know what I will do after that.

Simon Wadley

Nicola (18+) is still unsure of the way ahead. She had some very efficient surgery at the age of seven and can walk quite well. She attended a day special school (for physically handicapped children) and then moved on to a residential school where she is in the extended education unit,

learning the skills of daily living. Her next placement has
not yet been decided.

Peter is very severely handicapped and is totally dependent
for all his needs on those who care for him. His mother
writes the account of her fight for suitable facilities for him
and others as they leave school. The article from which
these extracts are taken was written in November 1985.

My son Peter is nearly 16 and has been at Rose Hill
School since it opened when he was five. We have two
other children, Caroline who is 18 and doing 'A'
Levels at High School and James, nearly 12, at a
Middle School. We have never expected anything of
them where Peter is concerned. We have always felt
that what they feel for him and what they choose to do
for him and with him must come from them and must
not be imposed. Happily, they are both loving and
caring and voluntarily take a share in entertaining and
caring for him. I hope that this philosophy will always
apply and that if the time comes when we can no
longer look after Peter, they will not be prey to
emotional blackmail to take over the responsibility.
This, coupled with the desire to do the best for Peter, is
why I am so anxious to secure Peter's future while I am
still here and able to fight for him.

When he was a baby, I heard a phrase on a radio
programme which stunned me and was to form the
basis of my philosophy of caring for Peter within the
family. It was that 'a family with a handicapped child
was a handicapped family'. Of course this is true but I
resolved there and then that this family would lead as
normal a life as possible and that Peter could only
benefit from having to fit into it. We were not going to
give in and allow our lives to revolve around him. I
think that those who know us well would say we have
succeeded. But we have only done it by sharing the
burden with the staff at Rose Hill and the relief care

service. As he gets older and bigger it is becoming more and more difficult to keep our heads above water and the days when I feel I just can't go on become more frequent.

We need an even greater level of support not less. And yet at a time when most parents of 16–18 year olds are looking to loosen the ties with their children, we are suddenly faced with the prospect of having to shoulder the entire burden. It is a devastating prospect. We just cannot do it. We have spent 16 years building a quality of life for Peter and for ourselves. Is anyone really going to be so cruel as to pull the rung out from under us?

In the early stages the only way I could cope was to get through one day at a time. To look back to the circumstances of Peter's birth and ask 'Why me?' only evoked bitterness and self pity, two negative and self-destroying emotions I have never been able to afford. Equally, the future was too terrifying and heart-breaking to contemplate. So I buried my head in the sand and got on with the job.

Then the day came when Peter's consultant paediatrician asked me what plans I was making for Peter's future and when I replied none, he said that I ought to start thinking about it because nobody would do it for me, and he implied that I would find that existing facilities were negligible. How right he was.

So I dragged my head out of the sand and started slowly and painfully to piece together my vision for Peter's future. This would be a local day centre where the educational and social programmes started at school would be continued and physio- and occupational therapy would be available. At the same place there would be a short term relief care facility which over the years would gradually increase until it became a long term care facility, and Peter would have a home which he knew and where he was known and cared for when we could no longer look after him.

Talking to other parents I began to realise that they shared my vision. This is what they, too, want for their children.

Imagine our horror and disappointment when we tried to fit the vision to the reality only to find that there is no reality. There is no adequate provision in this county for profoundly multiply handicapped school leavers, the most needy, the host helpless, the most dependent members of our society. Nothing!

The nearest we get to a vision of how society should incorporate its handicapped members comes from the Warnock Report. Integration is the key word. But how difficult it is to sustain a programme of integration when society's representatives, those who hold the purse strings, appear at best indifferent and at worst uncaring. Close the big hospitals and institutions and bring people out into the community—yes, good idea—saves money. Provide the community places— no, bad idea—costs money.

However, we parents and the education authorities accepted the challenge of Warnock. We have brought up our children in the community, taken them to church, to village fetes, to school functions, on outings and to the shops. We have begun the process of trying to change attitudes and to educate the general public into accepting them as members of the community. They have gone to school daily where each child has its own programme designed to stimulate and encourage that child to reach its potential. They are small steps measured against the achievements of normal children but, nevertheless, it is a quality of life. Best of all, they have the security of being surrounded by loving and caring people both at home and at school and they respond to that. To throw them on the scrap heap or to the mercies of exhausted and crumbling families at 19 negates and devalues the devoted and expert work of these people, and is nothing less than cruel to the children themselves.

All we are asking for is a continuation of that level of care, education and stimulation when they leave school. We are willing to go on sharing it for as long as we can, but the time has come for the balance to change. For our own health and sanity we have to start loosening the ties and preparing the children/young adults for the time when we can no longer go on caring for them at home. But we need to feel that their new home is secure and permanent, a place that they know and where they are known and cared for.

We are conscious of the fact that there are many more parents who find it difficult to speak for themselves and their children. We would like to speak for all of them and ask that provision be made for all school leavers who need it.

Postscript (November 1987)
This vision has been realised for Peter. A Special Day Unit for six severely handicapped young people has just been opened in his local area. They will attend every week day, and there will be two bedrooms available for respite or crisis stay in a place they know.

References

ANDERSON, E. M., CLARKE, L. and SPAIN, B. (1982). *Disability in Adolescence*. London: Methuen.

BRIMBLECOMBE, F. (1987). 'The voice of disabled young people —the Exeter Project', *Children and Society*, 1, 258–70.

COPE, C. and ANDERSON, E. (1977). *Special Units in Ordinary Schools*. London: University of London Institute of Education.

GLENDINNING, C., HIRST, M., BALDWIN, S., PARKER, G. and WARREN, L. (1987). *After 16—What Next?* York: Family Fund, Joseph Rowntree Memorial Trust.

HEGARTY, S. and POCKLINGTON, K. with LUCAS, D. (1981). *Educating Pupils with Special Needs in Ordinary Schools*. Windsor: NFER—Nelson.

MADGE, N. and FASSAM, M. (1982). *Ask the Children. Experiences of*

Disability in the School Years. London: Batsford Academic and Educational Ltd.

MORGAN, M. R. (1974). 'Like other school leavers?' in *The Handicapped Person in the Community*, pp. 222–224. BOSWELL, D. M., and WINGROVE, J. M. (eds). London: Tavistock Publications and Open University.

O'MOORE, M. (1980). 'Social acceptance of the physically handicapped child in the ordinary school', *Child: care, health and development*, **6**, 317–337.

SHEARER, A. (1974). 'Sex and handicap', in *The Handicapped Person in the Community*, pp. 225–227. BOSWELL, D. M. and WINGROVE, J. M. (eds). London: Tavistock Publications and Open University.

YOUNGHUSBAND, E., BIRCHALL, D., DAVIE, R. and PRINGLE, M. L. K. (1970). *Living with handicap.* London: National Bureau for Co-operation in Child Care.

Part Three

PROVISION OF SERVICES

9 Statutory Provisions

The worth of a State, in the long run, is the worth of the individuals composing it

John Stuart Mill

Bringing up a child who has a disability is an expensive process. It poses demands on the parents for time and patience, physical energy and determination, and often becomes a financial burden; for the child it challenges the whole personality, involving physical effort, intellectual response, courage and determination; from the community, practical support, interest and encouragement is called for, and the response comes from central and local government and from voluntary organisations.

Statutory sources promote a legislative framework through which public money affords finance and management for local services, some which must and others which may be provided. The details of how the mandatory services can be available are usually fairly flexible, so this accounts for the variability in the way such services are made available to children and their families. The usual facilities for the general population are an important factor in offering support for all types of disability, and additional services can also be provided.

Health Care
'On the ground' health care is provided by the District Health Authority which administers both hospital and community services.

Hospitals are largely concerned with acute and specialist problems. Maternity services, neonatal and special care units, in-patient and out-patient care, diagnostic facilities and often Child Development Centres are in the charge of hospital administrators and hospital health care staff, with a very close link with community services, particularly for children who need continuing care.

Community services have been rapidly developed under the NHS and expansion of their role is still continuing. For all children, particularly for those with persisting disability, they are of extreme importance, and it is worth considering this in some detail.

Health visitors, who work with family doctors, are the first line of contact for mothers of young babies. They make home visits regularly, advise about feeding, rearing, social training, minor behaviour problems, and keep notes on the baby's growth and development. Some are specially trained, and often based at the Child Development Centre, to support children who show developmental delay and their families.

Child health clinics Some GPs like to run their own children's clinics, others are established at health centres, manned by health visitors and supervised by specially trained Clinical Medical Officers. At these clinics parents can meet and compare their baby's progress. Weight and development are always recorded, immunisations can be administered, and advice on any problem is available from the health visitor or doctor.

School health is also an important function of the Community Health Service, and particularly so in special schools or in mainstream schools which are attended by children with 'special educational needs'.

Child Development Centres, whether situated in hospital, educational or voluntary premises, have important health contributions to the assessment and care of children who attend. The local 'District Handicap Team' is often based in these units, and community therapists may use them as their headquarters.

Liaison with local authorities, both education and social services, is clearly essential for all community activities. When this is successful, school nurses are seen as an integral part of the school, and teachers and social workers are at home in the Child Development Centre.

Artificial Limb and Appliance Centres (ALACs) are directly administered by the DHSS. These are regional centres, usually based in hospital grounds, which supply wheel-chairs of a suitable type requested by family doctors or hospital consultants, to children who need them. Calipers and artificial limbs also come under their jurisdiction.

All these services can combine to help the child and family to mix with other people in the community.

Social Services

Direct government help is supplied financially through a number of benefit schemes. Many of these such as *family allowance* and *supplementary benefit* are available to families without disabled members, although some factors related to the handicap may increase a teenager's eligibility for supplementary benefit.

However, there are allowances specially for handi-capped children and their families:

Attendance allowance is available from the age of two years for children who require attention or supervision during the day and/or night, which is very much more than would be needed for an able-bodied person of that age.

The *Mobility allowance* (Leaflet NI 211) is payable over the age of five years for children whose ability to walk is severely limited in distance, speed or manner, in compari-son with people of his own age.

Severe disability allowance is payable in some circum-stances to young people over the age of 16 years.

As the regulations for eligibility are often complex and may vary from time to time, it would be wise to consult your local Citizen's Advice Bureau, or National Insurance Office about making applications.

Government Sponsored or Funded Projects Administered by Other Bodies

Citizen's Advice Bureaux   These are situated in most towns, and are available to give free advice on all manner of subjects including government benefits.

The Family Fund is administered by the Rowntree Trust,

which offers financial help for holidays, domestic apparatus such as washing machines, and helps with other practical problems which are not covered by other benefits for needy families.

Local Provisions
Local authority social services are funded from the rates and are available to residents of a specific locality:

In the home, on the advice of occupational therapists, equipment for social needs can be supplied and home adaptations carried out such as the fitting of grab rails, downstairs toilets and showers, and sometimes chairlifts.

Outside the home, daytime facilities for young people such as Day Centres, where care is provided, or Adult Training Centres, where those with a mental handicap can find occupation, primary education, simple employment and training in social skills.

Residential facilities such as those described on pp. 131–2 and 144 can be provided by enlightened and pioneering social services departments.

Education
In Chapter 7 we discussed in some detail the educational services that may be required for children who have cerebral palsy, without indicating the administrative background. Central government enacts legislation, publishes advisory documents and sets standards. Local education authorities, funded largely by rates, support disabled children in mainstream schools, provide special schools where necessary and, in certain cases, may be responsible for fees for children in schools run by voluntary bodies. The Authority arranges for 'statements' to be made and discusses with parents and professionals the most suitable placement for each child. After school, children are supported in whatever form of Further Education that may be suitable for their ability.

10 Voluntary Organisations

A volunteer is worth two pressed men.

Anon

Voluntary organisations have been concerned with the care of disadvantaged children since the mid-nineteenth century. Many of these, e.g. Dr Barnado's, The Children's Society, National Children's Homes, are still actively involved and others have come into prominence more recently.

Some are local organisations, springing up in response to a local need or local branches of a national organisation which offers support and advice, or the national bodies themselves may take the initiative in organising activities or providing services. Whatever the source, close liaison with State provisions, whether in funding or professionalism, is of the greatest benefit to all.

The functions of voluntary organisations are very varied: (i) acting as a pressure group to local or central government for the provision of services or legislation to fulfil specific needs; (ii) dissemination of information to the public or to professional workers by using the media, publishing their own material or running conferences, courses and seminars; (iii) involvement in research, either by participating or by funding projects; (iv) training professionals in specific aspects of care; (v) setting up services and activities either locally or nationally.

The national organisations may concern themselves with children and/or adults with specific disabilities, or a mixture, and may or may not restrict their involvement to limited activities as in sport or education. Their contribution to the welfare of disabled children cannot be quantified, but certainly provides enrichment over and above the provision which the State is obliged or permitted to furnish. The voluntary sector has certain advantages over the more cumbrous functioning of the State. It is to experiment, to pioneer advances in management of children, to change the function and direction of units when the needs and demands alter. It tends to be more answerable to the voice of parents, and is able to make a direct appeal to the public for their interest and for funds.

The following pages give details of some of the national organisations which are of most relevance to cerebral palsy.

ASSOCIATION OF CROSSROADS CARE ATTENDANT SCHEMES LTD

10, Regent Place, Rugby, Warks CV21 2PN. Tel: 0788 73653

Crossroads exists to care for the carers, to help them to cope at home in looking after their disabled child or adult. Parents of very helpless children have a physically demanding task, with the need for constant attendance and often with broken nights, the need for turning the child, problems of incontinence, disturbed sleep patterns or frequent fits. The care attendant comes in at regular times and additionally at times of special need (in the daytime to allow Mum to get out for shopping or the hairdresser, in evenings so that Mum and Dad can have an evening out together, and sometimes overnight or at weekends). This kind of breather is often just enough to help the parents to keep going and to keep their disabled child at home.

Crossroads schemes have been established in more than 98 localities. They work very closely with social services, health authorities and local GPs, although they also accept direct referrals from the families themselves.

THE BRITISH SPORTS ASSOCIATION FOR THE DISABLED

Hayward House, Barnard Crescent, Aylesbury, Bucks HP21 9PP. Tel: 0296 27889

The Association caters for disabled people of any age and disability.

Its objectives are:

To be the co-ordinating body of sport and physical recreation for all disabilities. To encourage disabled people to take part in physical recreation and sport, for pleasure, for physical, emotional and social benefit, as an aid to rehabilitation, and to further opportunities for integration with the able-bodied community. To secure the provision and improvement of facilities for physical recreation and sport for disabled people by national and local government. To make more widely known the opportunities and the benefits to be gained from physical recreation and sport for disabled people.

Regional and national games are organised and teams are sent to international sporting events for the disabled; our British representatives often have much greater success than their able-bodied peers.

This is an organisation that can continue to provide leisure facilities for young people after leaving school or college, so long as efforts can be made on their behalf for continued participation.

CONTACT-A-FAMILY

16, Strutton Ground, Victoria, London SW1P 2HP.

Tel: 01-222-2695

This is a service which started in London but which is gradually extending throughout England. Its motto is 'a problem shared is a problem halved', and its aim is to put families in touch with others with similar problems. It does this mainly by help in setting up, monitoring and developing local groups. It has recently established a separate telephone line ('Contact Line' 01-222-2211), which is manned on weekdays from 10.30–14.30 by specially trained parents and volunteers, who, with background advice from their professionals, will be able to put callers in touch with another family with similar problems, or with someone who can guide them to local services available.

DISABILITY ALLIANCE

25, Denmark St., London WC2. Tel: 01-240-0806

(Publishes Disability Rights Handbook)

DISABLED LIVING FOUNDATION
  380/384, Harrow Road, London W9 2HU.
Tel: 01-289-6111

MOTABILITY
  The Adelphi, John Adam Street, London WC2N 6AZ.
Tel: 01-839-5191

NATIONAL BUREAU FOR HANDICAPPED
STUDENTS
  336, Brixton Road, London SW9 7AA. Tel: 01-274-0565
The Bureau was formed in 1976 to help young people with
any type of handicap to find the means to progress to
further, higher or adult education. It provides information
and advice for students and institutions through publications, seminars and conferences and through specialist
help and consultancy.

It can be especially helpful to young people considering
post-school educational placements; to careers staff in
education and social services, who have little experience of
a particular handicap and need guidance as to the possibilities for individual · students; and to institutions to
which pupils with adequate academic qualifications have
applied, but who may have additional needs for daily
living.

NATIONAL COUNCIL FOR SPECIAL EDUCATION
  1, Wood Street, Stratford-upon-Avon, Warwickshire
CV37 6JE. Tel: 0789 205332
The Council 'exists to further the education of *all* children
and young people with any form or degree of special
educational need, wherever they may be receiving care and
education. . . . It has always been chiefly concerned with
creating and fostering educational excellence and public
opinion for the disabled.'

It sees its function as a pressure group whose evidence is
sought in parliament, and as a focus for dissemination of
knowledge of good educational practice, and of advances

in educational techniques. It publishes its own practical guides, and monitors and recommends useful literature from other publishers.

As cerebral palsy is the cause of only a small fraction of special educational needs it is not always a chief focus of attention, but within the Council there exists a wealth of expertise on the subject.

NATIONAL DEAF CHILDREN'S SOCIETY
45, Hereford Road, London W2. Tel: 01-229-9272

NATIONAL PORTAGE AND HOME TEACHING ASSOCIATION
R. J. Cameron, Winchester Portage Service, Silver Hill, Winchester SO23 8AF

PHAB (Physically Handicapped and Able-Bodied)
Tavistock House North, Tavistock Square, London WC1H 9HX. Tel: 01-388-1963
PHAB celebrated its 30th Anniversary in 1987. Its aim is 'making more of life together' and it has been a pioneer in promoting social integration, particularly in leisure pursuits. It acts through local groups in forming clubs in which people meet together as equals to share common interests, and at national level organises holidays, camps and expeditions.

Increasing integration in schools may well encourage more integrated and exciting out-of-school activities in which PHAB clubs will play their part.

PLAY MATTERS (THE TOY LIBRARIES ASSOCIATION FOR HANDICAPPED CHILDREN AND ACTIVE)
68, Churchway, London NW1 1LT. Tel: 01-387-9592
PLAY MATTERS is the central organisation which links toy libraries which have been set up by local groups in response to local needs. These may be attached to hospitals (in children's wards or child development centres), to nursery schools, playgroups and day centres (whether voluntary or

run by local authorities). They may be separate facilities and sometimes are mobile, visiting children's homes.

The central organisation provides information, training and advice on suitable toys to those setting up toy libraries. ACTIVE is especially concerned with selection and production of toys for disabled children, usually with the support of physiotherapists and occupational therapists.

These libraries are extensively used, particularly for children disadvantaged in any way.

PRE-SCHOOL PLAYGROUPS ASSOCIATION (PPA)

61–3, Kings Cross Road, London WC1. Tel: 01-833-0991
The PPA is a national association which sustains, supports and advises local playgroups all over the country. These groups vary in size according to local needs, and take in children, usually aged three–five years. They have close links with the local social services and are subject to certain statutory obligations. The leader(s) receive training, organised locally by the PPA, and may receive a small salary. Mothers are encouraged to help at the group, which usually meets for two–three hours in a morning or afternoon. A small fee is charged for each child, who may not necessarily attend every day.

These groups are often the first opportunity for a disabled child to mix with able-bodied peers, usually in a ratio of 1:10. The association has published a very helpful booklet.

Opportunity classes, sponsored by the PPA, cater for a much higher proportion of handicapped children and need to involve more mothers in their day-to-day activities. They offer a stronger and more structured support service for parents.

QUEEN ELIZABETH'S FOUNDATION FOR THE DISABLED

Leatherhead Court, Woodlands Road, Leatherhead, Surrey KT22 0BN. Tel: 0372-842204
'Queen Elizabeth's Foundation for the Disabled, a

voluntary organisation, provides facilities for disabled men, women and young people from 16 upwards from all parts of the United Kingdom: assessment and further education; mobility centre; vocational training; sheltered workshop, arts centre and hostel; holidays and convalescence.' Of particular relevance to young people with cerebral palsy is Banstead Place, which offers assessment and further education for handicapped school leavers. The Foundation publishes an up-to-date Directory of Opportunities for School Leavers with Disabilities.

RADAR (THE ROYAL ASSOCIATION FOR DISABILITY AND REHABILITATION)

25, Mortimer Street, London W1N 8AB. Tel: 01-637-5400 RADAR may be looked upon as the power house and library for disabled people. It provides information on holidays and travel, sport and leisure, mobility, access, aids and adaptations, education, employment, welfare, training and rehabilitation.

It acts as a watchdog on new legislation, and in its fact-filled Bulletin, published each month, it ensures that its readers whether lay or professional (in many different disciplines) are kept up-to-date in all aspects of progress in medical, educational and social provision.

RIDING FOR THE DISABLED ASSOCIATION (RDA)

Avenue R, National Agricultural Centre, Kenilworth, Warks CV8 2LY. Tel: 0203 56107 Through local member groups RDA provides facilities throughout the country for disabled children and adults to ride (often in indoor riding schools).

The therapeutic value of riding for children who have cerebral palsy has been mentioned in Chapters 6 and 7, and most special schools for physically handicapped children arrange riding sessions for pupils during school hours. Children who attend ordinary schools may need to fit their riding in at other times. Parents or local groups may arrange this with the advice of the physiotherapist.

ROYAL NATIONAL INSTITUTE FOR THE BLIND
224, Great Portland Street, London W1N 6AV.
Tel: 01-388-1266.
Runs special schools for visually impaired children with other disabilities, including cerebral palsy.

SCOTTISH COUNCIL FOR THE WELFARE OF SPASTICS
22, Corstorphine Road, Edinburgh EH12 6HP.
Tel: 031-337-9876
The council is mostly concerned with providing services. It operates a Mobile Therapy Unit, based in Glasgow for children, mainly pre-school, but also those attending mainstream schools, in the west of Scotland. It runs three special schools, several work centres, and affords independent living accommodation in Perth and Edinburgh, working closely with local authorities and health boards.

THE SPASTICS SOCIETY
(Headquarters) 12, Park Crescent, London W1N 4EQ.
Tel: 01-636-5020.
(Social Services) 16, Fitzroy Square, London W1P 5HP.
Tel: 01-387-9571
The Spastics Society is concerned with all aspects of life for people who have cerebral palsy. It pioneers new ways of fulfilment and enrichment of life for people of all ages and all degrees of severity of disability. Its activities encompass all aspects of the work of voluntary organisations.

As a pressure group it has been active in encouraging education in mainstream schools, in campaigning for means of mobility, reasonable cash benefits, access to public buildings and for many other ways which may enable disabled people to take more part in community life.

In the dissemination of information, films and videos are produced for public use, pamphlets are available to parents and professionals on many subjects, and the scientific publications, the journal *Developmental Medicine and Child Neurology*, and monographs in the series *Clinics in Develop-*

mental Medicine, which are read all over the world, are respected for their authority and excellence.

Research The Society endowed the Prince Philip Chair in Paediatric Research, at Guy's Hospital, and also gives generous grants to research workers throughout the country to support research into many facets of the problems of cerebral palsy.

Training of professionals is carried out at Castle Priory College at Wallingford, through the organisation of seminars and courses, national and international, for the informed exchange and update of information. This is also promoted by the Medical Education and Information Unit at the Newcomen Centre at Guy's Hospital.

Setting up services for spastic people This may take the form of pump-priming and funding the building of units to be run locally by the Health, Social Services or Education authorities or by local spastics groups of which there are 180, or the Society itself may set up and run units, usually for special groups.

The Family Advisory Centre in Fitzroy Square offers assessment and advice to families; pre-school and nursery care is usually offered through local groups. In education, realising that not all children will be able to benefit from placement in mainstream schools, several residential schools have been organised for able children with severe or multiple disability, for less able children with behaviour problems, or for any groups which have special educational requirements which cannot be met in mainstream schools. Several of their schools and nurseries have adopted some of the principles of conductive education pioneered by Professor Peto in Hungary.

It is perhaps for its expanding facilities for those who have left school that the Society is most notable. Amongst these are: Beaumont College in Lancaster; workshops in various parts of the country; training centres and day centres; and residential units of many different types which cater for the various needs of the growing-up population of spastic people. Careers officers and social workers based at

Regional Headquarters are able to offer advice and support tailored to the needs of each individual. This is especially helpful for young people who are being catered for by local groups.

SPOD (THE ASSOCIATION TO AID THE SEXUAL AND PERSONAL RELATIONSHIPS OF PEOPLE WITH A DISABILITY)

286, Camden Road, London N7 0BJ. Tel: 01-607-8851/2
SPOD was founded as a voluntary committee in 1972 by a group of professional carers, who were concerned that the sexual needs and identity of people with a disability were being overlooked, ignored and denied.

It provides an advisory and counselling service for disabled people with sexual difficulties; an information service for professional and voluntary workers among the disabled; education and training on the sexual aspects of disability.

VOLUNTARY COUNCIL FOR HANDICAPPED CHILDREN

8, Wakley Street, London EC1V QE. Tel: 01-278-9441
This is an advisory service on all aspects of childhood disability. It is an independent council consisting of representatives nominated by professional bodies concerned with all aspects of care for children, and others elected by voluntary organisations concerned with a variety of disability in childhood.

The council's work is mainly strategic, commenting on government policy on the development of services for children, and proposing innovations in administrative procedures. The staff also deal with individual appeals for advice and guide enquirers to sources of help.

11 What of the Future?

Not all centres are able to provide the services that have been outlined in this book; further considerable resources will need to be made available before all have access to high quality services.

Part I of this chapter will consider some points for discussion on prevention of cerebral palsy, and Part II will deal with the needs for increase in services and some of the ways in which these might be provided.

PART I Prevention

Twenty years ago it was suggested that in the United Kingdom the incidence of cerebral palsy might be expected to decline, but in an investigation in Birmingham, comparing two consecutive five-year periods, Griffiths and Barrett (1967) found no significant change. Since then some workers (Stanley, 1979, in Western Australia and Hagberg and his co-workers in Sweden, 1975) have reported a decline in the incidence of cerebral palsy, although it appears that world-wide, where figures are available, most countries still show an incidence of approximately two to two and a half per 1000 live births (Paneth and Kiely, 1984). This situation, despite the improvement in maternity services and neonatal care that has occurred during this period, might suggest that no progress has been made, and that improvement in services has been ineffective in preventing cerebral palsy. More detailed consideration and investigation reveals two significant changes. Firstly, that there has been a decrease, almost to the point of elimination, of some types of cerebral palsy, and secondly, through the advance in the care of very small premature babies, there has been an increase in survival in this group

(Kitchen et al, 1979; Dale and Stanley, 1980; Hagberg et al, 1982).

Thus, at present there seem to be two groups of babies who are later recorded as having cerebral palsy.

In the first group are the premature babies, in particular those of low birth weight below 1500 grams. Modern methods in management in Special Care and Intensive Care Baby Units have enabled a much greater number of these vulnerable babies to survive, and whilst this means that there are many more living healthy normal babies who were very small at birth, equally there are more babies who survive yet have cerebral palsy. A considerable amount of research into the causes of brain damage in very low birth weight babies is taking place in various centres in the United Kingdom and around the world. Three methods of scanning brain structures are now available. Ultrasound, computer tomography (CT Scan), and magnetic resonance imaging (MRI), all show up the difference between normal brain tissue, haemorrhage, damaged tissue and cysts and indicate their location within the brain. By following up the survivors and recording their developmental progress it has become possible to find out which types and sites of damage have the most serious significance for the child's future. Thus, whilst it will become much easier to give firm reassurance much sooner to some parents, others may be presented with unfavourable expectations quite soon after the baby's birth, but this in the end may turn out to be easier to live with than continuing uncertainty.

In the second group are the bigger full-term babies, and in these evidence of perinatal and neonatal difficulties is found less often than previously. This has led Stanley and her co-workers (Dale and Stanley, 1980), to the conclusion that nowadays a higher proportion of severe cerebral palsy in full-term babies is due to either prenatal or genetic causes, which will be difficult to prevent. Much research will be needed to identify these.

At the present time it is difficult to be optimistic about the chances of preventing all causes of cerebral palsy in the foreseeable future, and this makes it all the more important to continue to improve existing and future services.

PART II Services
Here we are faced with a dilemma in trying to produce individual planned programmes for a small minority group of disabled people whose difficulties show great complexity and diversity. Some needs are common to all but individuals may require quite different means of fulfilment.

Research
In contrast to the widespread and detailed research that is possible into the factors that may be the cause of cerebral palsy, it is extremely difficult to plan valid controlled research into the efficacy of the many methods of helping. There are two major difficulties in the way: a) the near impossibility of finding a control series matched for all the other factors that may be relevant in contributing to a child's potential and progress; b) the extended time before it is possible to evaluate the effects of the methods used. Prospective studies can be fairly easily carried out to monitor the results of various kinds of brain damage detected by scanning, but it is a different ball game then to try to follow the relative merits of different ways of administering services. Retrospective studies need to be carried out on a large number of children, and the multiplicity of variables makes evaluation of individual factors in treatment and education almost meaningless.

In the long run it is perhaps most helpful to consider the common needs expressed by the parents of young children and later by the young people themselves, and then go on to consider how these may be fulfilled. Both research and experience have highlighted the desires of parents for information (given as early as possible in a way that they can understand); ways of involvement that will enable them to feel that they are acting to help their child (without the whole day being taken up by 'exercises' or 'stimulation'); choice in the way they accept help that is offered and in the education of their child (usually with an expressed preference for integration into mainstream schools); a worthwhile way of life for their children on leaving school (in education, training, employment or occupation, and in daily living skills); the prospect of suitable residential accommodation when they are no longer able to cope. Young people seek independence, which also entails work, education and leisure pursuits, recognition of them as 'persons' and not 'cases', and integration as far as possible into the community.

It is interesting to note in the lives of the young people who contributed to Chapter 8, the varied ways that their needs and wants are being fulfilled.

Once these needs and aspirations are understood, central and local government and voluntary societies can begin to consider how these needs can be met, and what resources will be needed to do so.

Throughout previous chapters the needs and aspirations of children, young people and their families have been discussed, and the ways in which these can be met have been considered. However, it is clear that services available are by no means uniform or comprehensive and that many readers will be saying 'Why isn't it like that for us?' Certainly we can none of us feel satisfied with the present situation. We need to go on seeking new ideas for practical measures in all fields, but a great deal could be done now to implement procedures which have already been shown to be helpful.

There would appear to be three factors which hinder progress:

1.   Lack of knowledge. Because cerebral palsy only affects a minority of the population, understanding of its implications tends to be limited, and very often professional and parental voices find it difficult to make themselves heard.

2.   Lack of conviction. New projects for handicapped children need to be promoted by professionals in response to parental pressure, but cannot progress in competition with other demands in the public sector without the strong

support of administrators. Voluntary societies may have the urge and commitment but can never have the financial capacity required to fund all the services required.

3. Lack of resources. Good practice is being carried out all over the United Kingdom but it is patchy, and to that extent ineffective. Given knowledge and conviction, implementation still cannot happen without adequate resources.

a) Better involvement of families
Families are the greatest asset that cerebral palsied children have but they need help and support.

(i) Professionals need to improve their ability to impart *information*, both at the top level from explanation of the condition and means to be taken to alleviate it, and at grass roots level by frequent simpler explanation and reassurance. Team work needs to ensure that information is consistent and reliable.

(ii) Practical help. Parents want to *do* something to help their child, and must always be given hope. More specialist training for physiotherapists and their deployment in the community would be a step forward. *Self-help groups* can be encouraged.

(iii) Consultation. Parents wish to choose and take part in decisions. It is easier to ensure that decisions are realistic when full information is given based on comprehensive assessment, and when parents have seen the results of practical help based on knowledge and experience of a wide choice of methods and techniques of treatment.

b) Education
As a result of the 1981 Education Act changes are taking place in the integration of cerebral palsied children into mainstream schools. Although this is not new—Jean (p. 128) and Ruth (p. 134) were 'integrated' more than 20 years ago—children with more severe physical handicaps, who may be in wheelchairs, are now being admitted to both primary and secondary schools when the building is suitable, often in the case of secondary schools, in special units.

It would be inappropriate to omit consideration of the role of Conductive Education (Hari and Tillerman, 1984; Cotton, 1974) in these developments. The concepts of 'orthofunction' and 'holistic' management describe an approach to the training of cerebral palsied children that all professionals in this country would endorse, and indeed aim to practise. Many units in this country have adopted some of the methods advocated by Professor Peto with some success, in particular in pre-school centres (Cotton, 1967; Seglow, 1984) and with some mentally handicapped children (Cottam, 1986). All agree on the effectiveness of this approach in the Institute in Budapest, but it has been our objective to make plain the immense variation in physical and mental ability in children who have cerebral palsy, and to refuse help to no one, whether they will walk or not. So that although we would wish to take advantage of much that is excellent, it is difficult to see how a full-blown Conductive Education programme will be cost-effective. We would much prefer to see all Health and Local Education Authorities with resources in fully trained staff to match the codes of good practice already well tried.

c)   A better way of life for young people
McKinlay (1987) stresses this as the most challenging aspect of cerebral palsy. There is no doubt from the experiences of young people quoted in Chapter 8, that opportunities are opening up for some, but this is not the universal experience (Brimblecombe, 1987). There is a great need for the expansion of facilities for further education, training, employment and leisure activities. Independent residential accommodation on the lines of the community described by Jan (p. 130) and some of the Spastics Society's bungalows at Tiptree and the Scottish Council for Spastics Units in Perth and Edinburgh for both single and married people will be increasingly wanted.

d)   'Hi Tech' and microtechnology
Both aids to communication and to daily living can be

expected from increased development along these lines. It is bound to be costly as equipment may need to be devised individually.

In summary, although considerable progress has been made in helping children and young people who have cerebral palsy, it cannot be said that all questions have been answered nor problems solved.

There are still great gaps in our knowledge and we need to find out more precise details as to the cause in every case and to devise further measures of prevention. Although much has been achieved in making full-term birth not only safer for the baby but more fulfilling for the mother and father, and in ensuring the survival of those born too soon, it may prove impossible to protect every vulnerable immature brain from harm. Thus more knowledge is needed of prenatal and genetic factors which are at present unidentified.

The provision of services for children and the encouragement of independent living for young people, wherever possible, demands additional resources in staff and facilities, which will require additional finance but, more importantly, knowledge and training and the will to accept the challenge.

References

BRIMBLECOMBE, F. (1987). 'The Voice of disabled young people— the Exeter Project.' *Children of Society*, 1, 58–70.

COTTAM, P. (1986). 'An approach for the mentally handicapped', in *Conductive Education. A System for Motor Disorders*. COTTAM, P. and SUTTON, A. (eds). Beckenham: Croom Helm.

COTTON, E. and PARNWELL, M. (1967). 'From Hungary: the Peto method', *Special Education*, 56, 7–11.

COTTON, E. (1984). 'Integration of disciplines in the treatment and education of children with cerebral palsy', in *Paediatric Developmental Therapy*, pp. 246–258. LEVITT, S. (ed). Oxford: Blackwell.

DALE, A. and STANLEY, F. (1980). 'An epidemiological study of cerebral palsy in Western Australia, 1956–1975. II: Spastic cerebral palsy and perinatal factors', *Developmental Medicine and Child Neurology*, **22**, 13–25.

GRIFFITHS, M. and BARRETT, M. (1967). 'Cerebral palsy in Birmingham', *Developmental Medicine and Child Neurology*, **9**, 33–46.

HAGBERG, B., HAGBERG, G. and OLOW, I. (1975). 'The changing panorama of cerebral palsy in Sweden, 1954–1970. I: Analysis of the general changes', *Acta Paediatricia Scandinavica*, **64**, 187–192.

HAGBERG, B., HAGBERG, G. and OLOW, I. (1982). 'Gains and hazards of intensive neonatal care: an analysis from Swedish cerebral palsy epidemiology', *Developmental Medicine and Child Neurology*, **24**, 13–19.

HARI, M. and TILLERMAN, T. (1984). 'Conductive education', in *Management of the Motor Disorders of Children with Cerebral Palsy*, pp. 19–35. SCRUTTON, D. (ed). Spastics International Medical Publications. Oxford: Blackwell Scientific Publications Ltd; Philadelphia: Lippincott.

KITCHEN, W. H., RICKARDS, A., RYAN, M. M., McDOUGALL, A. B., BILLSON, F. A., KEIR, E. H. and NAYLOR, F. D. (1979). 'A longitudinal study of very low-birthweight infants. II: Results of controlled trial of intensive care and incidence of handicaps', *Developmental Medicine and Child Neurology*, **21**, 582–589.

McKINLAY, I. (1987). 'A revision of the neurology and aetiology of cerebral palsy', *Association of Paediatric Chartered Physiotherapists Newsletter*, **44**, 4–10.

PANETH, N. and KIELY, J. (1984). 'The frequency of cerebral palsy: a review of population studies in industrialized nations since 1950', in *The Epidemiology of the Cerebral Palsies*, pp. 46–56. STANLEY, F. and ALBERMAN (eds). Spastics International Medical Publications Oxford: Blackwell; Philadelphia: Lippincott.

SEGLOW, D. (1984). 'A Pattern of Early Intervention', in *Paediatric Developmental Therapy*, pp. 76–87. LEVITT, S. (ed). Oxford: Blackwell.

STANLEY, F. J. (1979). 'An epidemiological study of cerebral palsy in Western Australia, 1956–1975. I: Changes in total incidence of cerebral palsy and associated factors', *Developmental Medicine and Child Neurology*, **21**, 701–713.

Index